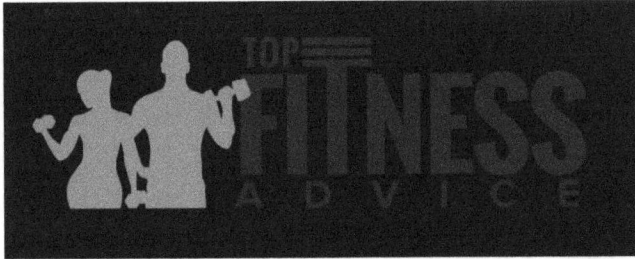

GET YOUR DREAM BODY

The EASIEST Way to Lose Weight FAST & Keep It Off FOREVER – You Have NEVER Tried A Weight Loss Plan Like This!

BONUS: Drop A Dress Size In 7 Days + Over 50 Recipes!

LINDA WESTWOOD

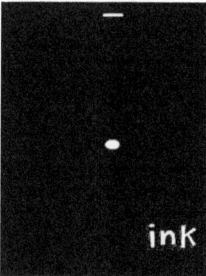

First published in 2015 by Venture Ink Publishing

Copyright © Top Fitness Advice 2019

Requests to the publisher for permission should be addressed to publishing@ventureink.co

For more information about the contents of this book or questions to the author, please contact Linda Westwood at linda@topfitnessadvice.com

Disclaimer

This book provides wellness management information in an informative and educational manner only, with information that is general in nature and that is not specific to you, the reader. The contents of this book are intended to assist you and other readers in your personal wellness efforts. Consult your physician regarding the applicability of any information provided in this book to you.

Nothing in this book should be construed as personal advice or diagnosis, and must not be used in this manner. The information provided about conditions is general in nature. This information does not cover all possible uses, actions, precautions, side-effects, or interactions of medicines, or medical procedures. The information in this book should not be considered as complete and does not cover all diseases, ailments, physical conditions, or their treatment.

You should consult with your physician before beginning any exercise, weight loss, or health care program. This book should not be used in place of a call or visit to a competent health-care professional. You should consult a health care professional before adopting any of the suggestions in this book or before drawing inferences from it.

Any decision regarding treatment and medication for your condition should be made with the advice and consultation of a qualified health care professional. If you have, or suspect you have, a health-care problem, then you should immediately contact a qualified health care professional for treatment.

No Warranties: The author and publisher don't guarantee or warrant the quality, accuracy, completeness, timeliness, appropriateness or suitability of the information in this book, or of any product or services referenced in this book.

The information in this book is provided on an "as is" basis and the author and publisher make no representations or warranties of any kind with respect to this information. This book may contain inaccuracies, typographical errors, or other errors.

Liability Disclaimer: The publisher, author, and other parties involved in the creation, production, provision of information, or delivery of this book specifically disclaim any responsibility, and shall not be held liable for any damages, claims, injuries, losses, liabilities, costs, or obligations including any direct, indirect, special, incidental, or consequences damages (collectively known as "Damages") whatsoever and howsoever caused, arising out of, or in connection with the use or misuse of the site and the information contained within it, whether such Damages arise in contract, tort, negligence, equity, statute law, or by way of other legal theory.

Table of Contents

Would you prefer to listen to my book, rather than read it?

Download the audiobook version for free!

If you go to the special link below and sign up to Audible as a new customer, you can get the audiobook version of my book completely free.

Go here to get your audiobook version for free:

TopFitnessAdvice.com/go/dreambody

Who is this book for?

Do you need a *strong* kick-start with your weight loss? Are you ready for a full body transformation in days, NOT weeks or months? Do you just wish that your fat would just fall off *effortlessly?* If you answered "Yes" to any of those questions – **this book is for you!**

I am going to share with you the most effective way to slim down and get flat abs, a firm butt and lean legs in just days! You are going to feel and look healthier than you have in years!

I have put it all together in this awesome book that will give you EVERYTHING you will need – from the theories, recipes, workouts, to the practical steps and action plans to implement the teachings in your life *immediately!*

The best part about is that you are going to see amazing results and this will *TRANSFORM YOUR BODY IN LESS THAN 3 WEEKS!* You can be a complete beginner or someone who works out regularly, it doesn't matter! If this sounds like it could help you, then keep reading...

What will this book teach you?

Inside, I will teach you many of the best ways to transform your body that will not only boost your weight loss, but also rejuvenate both your mind and body!

There are multiple sections in this weight loss system that you can utilize depending on what your individual goals are – that's what makes this book so awesome and effective at helping you lose weight! You will feel the healthiest you have ever felt – have the most energy you have ever had – and the fat will be melting *constantly!*

How? Because you're going to be eating well, and doing some of the most effective workouts that accelerates body transformation in a short period of time. PLUS, your plan is going to be specific to your individual goals, and the system is tailored in a way that boosts fat-burning all day and all night!

In this book, I give you the plan right in front of you that will change your life – all you have to do is follow it! One of the most important things for you to realize when reading this book is that it *really does work!*

However...

For you to achieve *real success*, you HAVE to apply this to your life. This is where most people fail – they read through the entire book but do nothing. You MUST try your best to apply as you read through the book!

Why will this book change your life TODAY?

This is a weight loss system that combines a low-fat, low-calorie, low-starch diet with targeted exercise, in order to deliver maximum results. Stick to the plan and follow the tips, and you will burn off fat, slim down, gain lean muscle, get fitter and become more toned all over.

It feels great to achieve our best body before we go on a vacation or when we want to enjoy the warmer months. It's a huge self-esteem booster to be able to wear summer clothes and look better than ever! Any even if you're not going on vacation or summer has already passed, there's nothing stopping you from looking sexy all the time!

Naturally, the benefits of this plan are not restricted to how you will look afterwards; they are also firmly focused on your health and how great you will feel. This is not a crash-diet – you will be losing weight steadily and in a healthy way without starving yourself, which means the results will ideally last FOREVER.

Finally, you are giving your body a great energy boost by engaging in exercise routines – both cardio and toning workouts – that are specifically chosen to nourish your mind and body. If you follow the plan, you will speed up your metabolism, improve your heart health, strengthen your bones and muscles, cleanse your digestive system, and boost your immunity. All that AND a great body! Time to get started...

Introduction

If you have been looking around for the best way to lose weight and drop a few dress sizes within the shortest period of time, this book is the one! A lot of research went into the creation of this book – so you don't have to waste time sifting through scientific results, expert opinions, and mainstream gossip about the "best practices" when it comes to weight loss. The hard job has been done for you, and I have put everything that you need to know *right here* in this short book!

Before you begin, I want to explain one important component of successful weight loss – probably the MOST important component. With all the garbage that is online and on TV promising "rapid weight loss" and how you can "lose 50lbs in 5 days", it's no wonder you are likely struggling with your weight loss. You are overwhelmed with so much in front of you that you have no idea what plan or diet you should do! Let me simplify this for you. In fact, if you only get one thing out of this book, please let it be what I'm about to say now. **Weight loss is simple. It's not easy, but it's simple. It's as simple as following a set plan. And at the core of the set plan lies one all-important fact, burn more energy than you consume.**

In this book, you are going to join me in creating the ultimate plan for you to follow – that is set by you and your limits, your capabilities, and your level of fitness – so that you will successfully lose weight. You are going to have a plan that you are GUARANTEED to follow. Why? Because it's going to be created and set by you.

How many times do you try a new weight loss plan or diet that is created by someone else, only to fail miserably within the first week (if you even make it past 3 days)? The main reason this happens is because it is either 1) too extreme for you as a beginner, and so you become overwhelmed and just stop, or 2) the plan or diet itself is plain GARBAGE – the amount of times I have come across "diets" that are nothing more than how-to guides on starvation and malnutrition is astounding! These things just encourage your body to go into starvation mode and drastically slow down your metabolism. The scariest part is that once your metabolism slows down, it is VERY hard to increase it again without implementing an effective plan that slowly speeds it up with the right foods and exercises.

In this book you are going to come across various sections. The first section is going to emphasis and focus on diet and food. Why? Because it's the most important aspect of weight loss. If it came down to either eating healthy or exercising daily, and you could only do one, eating healthy will lead to more weight loss than exercising and eating garbage. Obviously, if you can combine both, you are effectively *increasing* how fast you can lose weight. I have also included a section on the theory of weight loss, and how to successfully understand the lifestyle factors to guarantee success. A core part of this is understanding what makes up the food you eat, and by understanding just this simple thing, you can have a greater chance of success.

Finally, I have included a section on exercising and working out. You will learn what exercises are best to do if you're short on time and need the highest calorie burn. You will also find out what exercises to do in order to tone up certain areas of your body, such as your butt, thighs, belly, or arms. And, because I am really passionate about helping you lose weight and achieve your goals and dreams (plus all my fans have asked me to include this), I have added a final BONUS section that will teach you exactly how you can drop a dress size in 7 days. Simply follow the plan I have written, and you will be able to do it. It could not be any easier!

The 7 Reasons Your Previous Diets Have Failed!

This weight loss system is primarily based on providing what other diets and weight loss plans don't, which is why other diets fail and this has a greater rate of success! Below are seven of the main reasons why most diets fail, but not only am I going to explain them, I am going to give you an action plan on how to combat each one while you start this system!

1. You Get Hungry

This is one of the most common reasons why most diets fail – you get hungry. The truth is that it's not because you aren't eating enough – well, sometimes it is, especially if you're on a crash diet of some sort. Rather, it's more about eating the right macronutrients. This is how you are going to be able to apply it to your life. There are three main macronutrients; carbohydrates, fats and protein.

Unfortunately, most diets will focus on carbohydrates as the main source of calories – why? Because carbs contain the least amount of calories (same as protein) and can be digested the quickest.

Here are the numbers:

- 1 gram of fat contains 9 calories
- 1 gram of protein contains 4 calories
- 1 gram of carbohydrates contains 4 calories

Right there you can see that fat contains the most calories, and because most diets nowadays are focused on restricting calories, they all don't recommend consumption of fats. In terms of protein vs. carbohydrates, the truth is this. The primary sources of protein include meats, poultry and seafood. Unfortunately, a lot of protein sources also contain large amounts of fat and so the calorie counts increase. This is why many low-calorie diets are comprised of more carbs, percentage wise, when compared to protein and fat. That being said, here's what you need to focus on...

You need to find lean sources of protein – things like turkey, salmon, lean meats, chicken breast, etc. These all contains large amounts of protein but also very little fat, and barely any carbs. The reason I focus highly on protein here is because there's a secret with protein. It will burn anywhere from 25-30% of the calories it contains just through digestion. That means you are already burning off some of the calories from the food (if it contains large amounts of protein) while you're digesting it.

Additionally, this means you are going to feel full for a much longer time and LESS hungry! This is why diets fail; carbs don't keep you full long enough, and result in you eating more!

2. You Start Feeling the Power of Cravings

Another reason why many diets fail is because of cravings. Here are my best solutions to cravings that nearly always work:

- Avoid sugars and carbs as much as possible in the latter stages of the day. Once you start eating carbs, you usually crave more carbs; it's just how our bodies work. In fact, if you can try not to consume any carbs after 6pm, or if you're really committed, 3pm, this will be a huge help. Those cravings should cut in half, especially if you're one of those people who get most of their cravings at night!

- The second solution that always works for me is mint! When I am craving something, I will either start chewing on a piece of sugar-free chewing gum, or even better, brush my teeth! Seriously, try it next time you feel a craving coming on, and in within minutes you will notice the difference. Just think about how hungry you are immediately after brushing your teeth in the morning.

3. You Feel Restricted by Your Diet

This is a very common failing point of dieters and the best way to address this is to follow the system in this book. The truth is that no diet should ever cause you to feel restricted, and if it does, then it's not the right one for you. Using the methods in this weight loss system, and my recipes below, you will definitely notice that you feel *less restricted*, because you are STILL allowed to have many tasty, sweet foods!

4. The Diet Isn't Realistic for Me!

How many times have you thought that a diet looks great on paper but when it comes to the practical side of things it's just so difficult for you to implement it? Maybe you don't have access to the foods you need? Maybe you don't have a blender for the smoothies? Maybe you can't do the workouts you need to do while on the diet? Whatever the case is, this is a very common reason that most diets fail and it's understandable.

That's the great thing about this weight loss system - it's simple! It's easy to implement and can be done by anyone in the comfort of their own home! It will also be a great help if this is something that you struggle from because I will give you the actionable steps that will allow you to take the theory and apply it in your life.

5. Diets Are Boring!

This is definitely the leading reason I would fail with diets! I personally find them very boring, but then I realized something... The main reason they are boring is because I think of them as a restrictive plan that I am only going to follow temporarily. This is the wrong approach and mindset; in fact, this is the type of approach that would lead to me putting the lost weight back on at some point in the future. This is something that this weight loss system also addresses and looks to change. Its goal is to provide a plan that you don't feel is restrictive, so at the end of the day you are less likely to feel that it's a boring diet.

6. There Are Too Many Temptations

Again, this is yet another reason why diets fail that links to the entire idea that a diet is a restriction and not a long-term lifestyle change. When this is the case and the perspective, anyone on a diet is going to obviously get tempted by foods that they feel they are "restricted" from. That just leads to cheating in the diet, or the temptation gets to strong that you finally give in. Just like was suggested for the few previous issues, you need to get out of this "restrictive diet" mode and then you will see longer term success.

7. You Don't Get Good Enough Results

If you're not getting solid results you're going to end up feeling dissatisfied and it will lead to you quitting your weight loss plan. This can be solved by actually beginning a weight loss plan that will WORK – like the system in this book you are reading!

Discover Scientifically-Proven "Shortcuts" & "Hacks" to Lose Weight FASTER (With Very Little Effort)

For this month only, you can get Linda's best-selling & most popular book absolutely free – *Weight Loss Secrets You NEED to Know*.

Get Your FREE Copy Here:

TopFitnessAdvice.com/Bonus

Discover scientifically-proven tips to help you lose weight faster and easier than ever before. With this book, readers were able to improve their weight loss results and fitness levels. So, it's highly recommended that you get this book, especially while it's free!

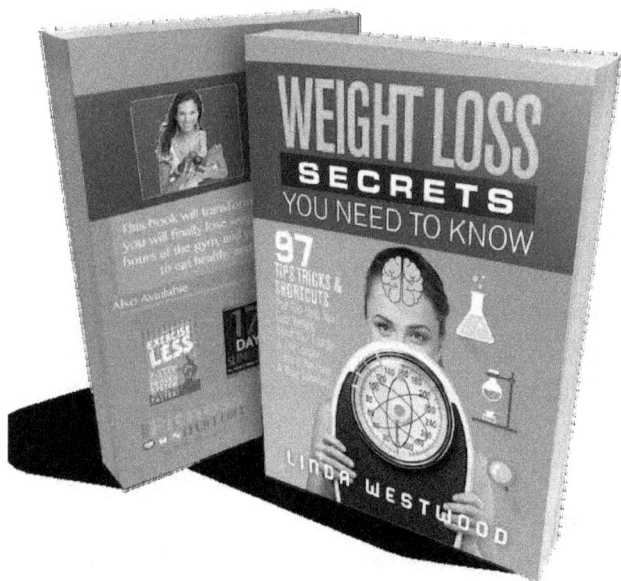

Get Your FREE Copy Here:

TopFitnessAdvice.com/Bonus

The Difference Between This Book & Others

There are two main differences between this weight loss book and others. Firstly, as I mentioned above, it doesn't focus on a temporary diet fix. Rather, it's a transitional program that aims to take you from where you are now to a full lifestyle change that has you losing weight and living healthy. As I mentioned above, many diets fail because they are restrictive and this leads to temptations, getting bored, feeling restricted, etc. In the creation of this weight loss system, the goal was to avoid these reasons and ensure that the same thing did not happen here as well. For this reason, my book is different.

The foods you learn about, and weight loss plan I share with you in this book are not "secret". They are not "magical" formulas. In fact, some of the foods aren't even full meals. They are simply the building blocks that are not only great for promoting weight loss because of their acceleration properties (more on this later in this step), but they can also be easily applied to your life. For this reason, I have included a quick-start guide to the beginning and broken it up into sections that make your weight loss a walk in the park, rather than a tough restrictive-focused diet.

Now, the second and main reason why this book really works and is different from the others, is because the foods that are promoted contain either thermogenic properties or are high in protein and fat, both of which I discuss in more detail. Additionally, the workouts have been scientifically proven to stimulate fat loss at a greater level than regular cardio workouts, such as walking, jogging, or cycling.

Finally, I have worked closely with over 150 overweight individuals and collated the most common reasons that they feel diets are difficult, why they fail to lose weight, what stops them from exercising, and several other key questions, and devised a solution which I present as tips at the end of this book! Going back to foods, let's take a look at thermogenesis closer. What is it? Thermogenic foods essentially boost your metabolism. That's the simplest explanation and really as much as you need to know if you're a beginner when it comes to this. Therefore, consuming highly thermogenic foods will not only satisfy hunger, but also keep you fuller for longer, and boost your metabolism – leading to more calories burned throughout the day whether you're resting or working out.

A rise in your metabolism (rise in your basal metabolic rate), will mean that your calories burned at rest also increases. There is science behind this, and that's why the foods and recipes I include are highly focused, in fact, based on foods that contain some sort of additional property, such as thermogenesis. So, remember that instead of trying to use your willpower to eat right and workout regularly, you have science on your side and can be burning more calories all day long!

Now, the added benefit of some of these foods, mainly the ones that don't contain as great of a thermogenic property as others, is that they are either high in protein or in fats, or in both. The digestion of protein will burn approximately 25-30% of the calories that it contains, where as to digest carbs you may only burn around 9%. For this reason, some of the foods recommended contain large amounts of protein.

Fats are also beneficial in this aspect, not only for the digestion, but also because fats keep you full for a long time too (just like protein)! This is because they are digested a bit slower because they need to get broken down. So, as you can see, this weight loss system focuses on a lot more than just calories and exercising, but rather these additional benefits of eating the *right* foods to promote weight loss as well as satisfy hunger, as well as looking at where the common weak points in diets are and fixing them!

Full Body Transformation – Kick Starter Program

This section will look at and present to you the best way to begin your weight loss journey – including some of the common questions that beginners encounter. You will get a three-phase weight loss program to get you started on your journey, and I will include 20 highly thermogenic and fat-melting foods that you can add into your life. And as a bonus, I have even thrown in a few recipes that include these foods!

Phase 1: The First 5 Days

Before we begin, realize that the goal of these 5 days is to transition successfully into what is considered a "lifestyle change" and not a "restrictive diet". You can do this by not focusing on what you CAN'T have, but rather the many things you CAN have.

Drinking Water Is Crucial

In this initial phase, one of the most important bits of knowledge should be that many of the times you feel hungry, you are actually thirsty. For this reason, you should always keep some sort of water with you, whether it's a bottle or a cup. Always stay hydrated, and be sure to start drinking more water in your daily life in these 5 days – this will help curb your hunger, but you will also benefit from some of the great things that more water in your life will give you.

1. Drinking enough water every day will allow your body to maintain its balance of fluids. Remember, your body is comprised of approximately 60% water. You need to ensure that your body has enough water because it's crucial to functioning.

2. Water WILL help you control the amount of calories you intake through food. As mentioned before, many of the times you think you're hungry, you're actually thirsty. Not only will this mean you eat less, but also because you're constantly topping up and staying hydrated, you will be less hungry throughout the day and need less "snacking moments".

3. Your muscle cells contain a lot of water and need water for effective and efficient functioning. This is another great benefit of water. You will feel less exhausted and your muscles will function much better!

4. A final benefit of water, which I believe is one of the best, is in relation to your skin. Water helps keep your skin looking fresh, clear and hydrated. This is because your skin also contains a lot of water - if you're dehydrated I'm sure you will know by feeling your skin.

Adjusting to A New Macro Balance

Once you start eating thermogenic foods you will obviously notice a great difference. That being said, your body will need to get used to it because right now you could be consuming any balance of macros. The recipes I include allow a greater proportion of your daily calories to come from protein and this change in balance is something that you will get adjusted to, both inside and outside.

Outside? Really? Yes! You need to learn what foods contain larger amounts of protein, so you can make great selections throughout your entire diet and life. And you will also start learning some great recipes that promote these properties of food. The best part about Phase 1 is that you aren't trying to eat all the foods at once. You are aiming to make some of the minor changes first, and then gradually through the other phases you can introduce other foods.

Do I Need to Work Out?

If you want to work out in this phase, you can, however the primary goal in this phase is to eat right. It's to focus on good foods and ensure that you're giving yourself the best possible chance of succeeding, and this is with the diet first!

Remember, approximately 80% of weight loss will be determined through your diet and what you eat on a daily basis, not the 30 minutes you put in at the gym (don't get me wrong though, working out is fantastic and will be added later in this process!).

So How Can You Apply Phase 1 In Your Life TODAY?

Now that you understand fully what Phase 1 is about and how you're meant to apply it, here are some actionable steps to get you started.

1. Understand what you are trying to do in this phase, and what your goals are. This is personal and up to you, however, I can suggest that an initial goal should be to focus on your diet in this phase, *and ONLY your diet!* I also suggest that you keep your goals short for this phase – one is perfect! Why? Because if you have any more than one, you run the risk of getting distracted, or even worse, not reaching all your goals in the initial stage will may leave you feeling dissatisfied and wanting to quit before you have even given yourself a chance!

2. Realistically, you can eat any thermogenic foods in this stage, it really doesn't matter, however there are certain recipes that are more recommended, and these are easier to prepare in the initial stages. For this reason, I have included my top 15 thermogenic recipes below!

3. The last step is to simply try and learn as much as you can! It's great that you're reading this book, but also go further and check out some other articles and blogs online that you

can learn from. Knowledge is power when it comes to weight loss, and there is nothing stopping you from learning exactly how you can transform your body and your life.

Remember, this is a learning phase, so there's nothing better than to actually learn the science and nutrition behind this diet so you can maximize and gain the most from it!

Phase 2: The Next 5 Days

This phase focuses on the next 5 days and how you can incorporate better foods into your life. Ideally, in this phase you should notice feeling more energetic throughout the day, waking up happier, and seeing / feeling a noticeable difference in your weight loss. How? By throwing more thermogenic foods into the mix.

Focus of Phase 2

One of the major changes here that you will be trying to make is to add the overall nutritional benefits that you need into your daily foods. The recipes, at this phase, will aim to focus on providing you with all the vitamins and minerals you need throughout the day via each meal. You can also start adding in a small workout at this point, but again it's up to you.

As with the previous step, diet is essential and the most fundamental part of the kick starter program. If you messed up your diet for a day, but did a great 30-minute workout, it's not as great as if you did AWESOME with your diet but forgot to workout. Remember, diet comes first.

Eating During Phase 2

In terms of the foods you will be eating during Phase 2, all thermogenic foods are open to your choice. There are many more recipes at this stage that become available to you which are suggested, and I cover these in my top 15 recipes below as well! You will notice that in this phase of the kick starter program the recipes that are suggested will be a mix of meals, snacks and even smoothies! This gives you a lot more variety – keeping in mind that variety is crucial so you don't feel bored or want to quit your diet because you feel it's too restrictive.

The recipes, generally, will contain at least two thermogenic foods, along with some sort of protein source. This will keep you full (the protein), while increasing your metabolism (the thermogenic ingredients). Ultimately, this is the best way to go about losing weight, and definitely one of the easiest ways to transition into a long-term lifestyle change. One final recommendation is that you leave the four hours spacing between meals as is.

So How Can You Apply Phase 2 Into Your Life?

Here are some actionable steps that you can take during Phase 2:

1. Take a look at your goals from Phase 1. How did you go? You need to analyze your results and measure whether or not you succeeded. If you succeeded, then that's great! If not, then you need to ask yourself why, and be honest about your answer because it will apply in this phase too.

2. Now I want you to make new goals for this phase. If you did well with one goal from the previous phase, then you can go one better and set yourself two goals here.

3. Keep learning and working on your diet. Make sure you're eating the right foods that are recommended in this book or if you find a larger list online. Also, now that you are encouraged to increase your thermogenic food intake, you can start changing up some recipes, leading to more variety,

or pick some of your favorite foods that you can always rely on to get you back on track.

4. Finally, keep learning and applying new things that you learn about this diet. The great part is that in the next phase, because it's longer, you will be able to add a lot more actionable steps to the mix and this will lead to great results. But until then, keep learning and focusing only on your diet. This is why this phase is also only 5 days, like the previous one, whereas the next phase is 21 days!

Phase 3: The 21 Days That Guarantee Weight Loss

This is the final phase of the kick starter program, but remember it doesn't mean it's the end. The kick starter program focuses only on 31 days so that you don't get overwhelmed. Realistically, I want this kick starter program to help you get your mindset focused on healthy living, and then you can continue onto the actual weight loss system that guarantees long-term success.

Focus of Phase 3

This phase focuses on taking the entire "diet" and turning it into a "lifestyle" change. You want to focus on steady weight loss throughout this entire phase and onwards past this phase until you reach your own fitness or weight loss goals. You will also learn how to eat when dining out, so that you don't end up breaking the success that you have thus far with the kick starter program.

Finally, you will have an even greater variety of foods that are encouraged in various recipes; this is also included in my top 15 recipes below!

Noticing the Changes

At this point you have been doing the kick starter program for over a week and so you should be noticing some fantastic changes with your body. If these changes are in the mirror, then that's great! However, where most of the changes are noticed at this stage is inside your body. You should be feeling a lot more energetic after ten days of the kick starter program! Not only that, but you should also be sleeping better and your overall body functioning should be a lot more effective and efficient in your everyday work.

Eating During Phase 3

During this phase you will be introduced to a LOT more recipes and meal plans that incorporate multiple thermogenic foods, as well as various sources of proteins. This is great because it presents you with more variety, and it's something that makes everything easier in the long-term. Remember, the focus of this phase is so you can maintain your weight loss and factor in for many of life's natural occurrences and events – such as dining out, or going out for drinks.

When dining out, you should focus on protein. Now that you know the great benefits of protein, you should be selecting meals that don't contain many carbs, but have great servings of protein. For example, a lean steak would be perfect! And, instead of having a side of fries with it, substitute it for a salad! This would be a great example of a meal that is perfectly fine to have when dining out during Phase 3. It contains a source of protein, minimum carbs, and a good variety of healthy salads.

Working Out During Phase 3

Hopefully by this phase you actually know a lot more about the fundamentals of foods; things like why protein is so beneficial to your body, and which foods are more thermogenic than others (contained in the foods section). Since your diet has hopefully made some great progress up to this point, you can now focus a little more on working out. Things like walking are great to begin with.

Why? Because it's simple and you can't really do too much wrong. I suggest that, if you're a complete beginner to working out, you start walking daily. The best part about it is that you can start with just 15 minutes a day, and then progressively walk more and more, until you get to a nice, brisk 45 minute walk every day. Not only is walking a great piece of cardio, which strengthens your heart, but it's also a milder workout that will focus more on fat burning in the long run. It's what our bodies were meant to do!

If you're someone who likes to go to the gym, then you're probably a little more advanced. You can try things like running, the stationary bike, or even the elliptical trainer. Any form of cardio is great, and if you're sweating and breathing harder than normal, then you're making progress in the right direction. Just remember, don't push yourself too hard!

Resistance Training

Since we're talking about working out, I have to point out that resistance training is something that you should definitely consider. You can do this through some simple weight training, even just lifting an extra pound or two is fine.

The benefits of resistance training are many:

- Your muscles and joints will become stronger, allowing for better functioning and movement. This is also correlated to longevity and health in older age.

- Resistance training helps tone your body, especially in those flabby areas, like your arms or belly. Arm workouts and abdominal workouts work great for those areas, respectively.

- One of the final and, in my opinion, best benefits of resistance training is the fact that it increases your metabolism for anywhere from 12 to 34 hours after you have finished your workout. This "afterburn effect" is great because along with your thermogenic diet, it will result in even faster weight loss!

So How Can You Apply Phase 3 In Your Life?

Below are my actionable steps to applying the Phase 3 to your life:

1. As with the previous step, look over your goals once again and see how you have been performing thus far in terms of achieving your goals. The reason I stress this as being important is because we are going to make some goals in this phase that will apply and stick with us for the rest of this phase and for the rest of our weight loss journey until we achieve them. So, if you find that there's a consistent area that you keep failing in, you need to ask yourself why and try to figure out how you can sort it out.

2. Now, make new goals, not only for this phase, but also for the rest of your journey. Remember, this is the phase that you aim to try and maintain your weight loss during. So if you have a lot of weight to lose, this is the phase that you need to set it as a goal, and focus on it daily.

3. In terms of eating, we are open to any thermogenic foods, as well as a variety of different protein sources. There are some great recipes in this book that will provide you with consistent results and a long-term plan of variety so you

don't get bored. Don't forget to continue focusing on your thermogenic foods as well because they do provide a great foundation of raising your metabolic rate – hence speeding up the entire weight loss process. Finally, when going out, make sure you opt for foods that provide a great source of protein, and minimize any carbohydrate intake. Also, add those spices and other thermogenics whenever possible.

4. Thankfully, in this phase we can also begin looking at working out. I suggest that you start walking every day for at least 15 minutes, depending on your current fitness levels. Walking is great and its benefits are endless and will contribute to your healthy life for many, many years to come. Also, remember to increase your activity levels at least once a week, so that you are not only improving your muscles, heart and overall body's fitness levels, but also because once you start losing weight you will need to work out that little bit extra to continue losing at the same rates.

These are the best ways that you can apply the three phases of the kick starter program into your life in the easiest way possible that allows for a transition from it being a "diet" into it being an amazing "lifestyle change". The final section of the kick starter program is focused on providing you some ending words of advice and tips that will not only make things easier for you, but also help you take your weight loss progress to the next level.

Accelerate YOUR Transition from The Kick Starter Program

These are some final bits of advice that will help you speed up your weight loss and take full control of your life in the long-term. This is especially important in transitioning from the kick starter program to the full weight loss system you will learn in this book!

Why You're Overweight

The truth is that, unfortunately, most people *believe* they are overweight because they are using food normally, but just not the right foods. However, this is incorrect. The real reason that most people are overweight is because they actually *misuse* foods in general. They don't know or understand how to use food appropriately in a way that will not only allow them to live a much healthy and prolonged life, but also one that promotes weight loss.

Takeaway Message: Aim to avoid eating food for any other reason than its nutritional benefits and purpose to provide fuel to your body.

Increasing Your Metabolism Is Crucial

Another important part of the kick starter program is that you *must* always look to increase your metabolism. With an increased metabolism, not only are you burning more calories at rest, but you are also burning more calories when you're working out. This is exactly why the foods are centered around thermogenesis.

Takeaway Message: Stick to foods that will help boost your metabolism. This is going to be a key contribution to your long-term weight loss success because it will provide a higher base level of calories burned daily.

It Comes Down to You, Your Mind & Your Body

At the end of the day, succeeding with weight loss comes down to you, your thoughts and your actions. No one is going to *make* you lose weight, and there is no magical cure. You need to fully *believe* that no matter what you ARE going to lose weight and ARE good at losing weight in the long run. You also need to believe that *you are a healthy person who is meant to live a healthy life.*

Takeaway Message: Thoughts and beliefs that are positive will lead to actions that reinforce those ideas – and THAT'S where the real success lies!

Don't Believe Fake Hunger

Another great tip is that our bodies naturally present thirst in a similar way that it presents hunger. For this reason, unfortunately, many people get trapped into thinking that they are hungry when, in fact, they are thirsty. This entire process repeats itself every day and before you know it you have eaten an insane amount of calories for no reason or nutritional value for the week and this is why you're putting on weight.

Takeaway Message: So instead of eating next time you feel this way, just drink a big glass of water instead. Nine times out of ten you will feel fine right after this, but if you're still hungry after a big glass of water, then definitely have a healthy snack!

Goal Setting Will Make You a Winner

One of the last and most effective tips that will help you achieve long lasting weight loss success is to set goals. Why? Because you can't win a race if you don't even know where or what the finish line is. I highly suggest setting goals and regularly assessing your progress and success. You can do this weekly or monthly.

One other great reason for goal setting is because of the motivation that it will bring to your whole journey of weight loss. You should always be focusing on your goals every day and taking steps towards the final goal every single day. I personally try to take at least one step toward my final goal every day, and won't sleep without taking at least one step toward my goals.

Takeaway Message: Set goals! Measure your progress regularly and make sure that you focus on them daily and use them to motivate you. This will increase your chances of success ten-fold.

I hope that you are enjoying this book so far, and if you could spare 30 seconds, I would greatly appreciate you leaving a review on Amazon.com.

The BEST Thermogenic Foods

I guess the biggest question that you probably want answered first is – what are the best thermogenic foods, and why exactly are they so great? Well, I have broken the up into categories below, so take a look:

Foods that have thermogenic effects and will burn fat when eaten

- **Coconut oil**: proven through various testing that the body will take the energy from coconut oil into the liver and use it almost immediately. This reduces storage of any of the energy into glycogen, or even fat. Also, coconut oil is made up of medium chain triglycerides that are shown to boost individual's metabolisms.

- **Green tea:** this one is so common nowadays that you probably already know about it. Green tea firstly contains caffeine, which is a stimulant and will boost your metabolism. Secondly, and more importantly, green tea contains epigallocatechin gallate, which is a substance that is proven to increase thermogenesis within your body.

- **Mustard:** the thermogenesis effect from mustard primarily comes from its added spice. Your body gets a slight metabolic shock when you consume spice and it will boost your metabolism.

- **Walnuts:** similar to mustard, the thermogenic effect from walnuts may only last a few hours after consumption, but considering the high healthy fat content, this will fill you up and provide your body with many benefits outside of weight loss too!

- **Olive Oil:** similar to walnuts, olive oil contains that same types of fats and has a likewise thermogenic effect that last for a few hours after consumption. Keep in mind this isn't just any oil, but olive oil in particular.

Foods that are going to keep you feeling FULL the longest

- **Almonds:** these are, by far, the most healthy and best nuts that you can consume. Not only are almonds proven through various studies to keep you feeling fuller for longer, but they also provide your body with many other benefits, such as lowering your cholesterol!

- **Apples:** these are the best fruits you can eat. Why? Because they are full of fiber and will keep you full for a *long time!* Not only that, but they have *also* been shown to reduce cholesterol when eaten regularly!

- **Yogurt:** if you choose the right type of yogurt, it can be very healthy for you. You need to look for a low-fat yogurt, but also check the nutrition table to ensure it's low in sugar as well. High in protein and antioxidants, yogurt will provide your body with some flavor and can be added into various smoothies and shakes!

- **Chickpeas:** this just comes down to the science; chickpeas are full of both protein and fiber, as mentioned previously, the two power substances in foods! They are going to keep you feeling full the longest, and also benefit your body in many other ways like heart health.

- **Cod:** the effects of cod are great, primarily due to its high protein content. This is linked to great body health as well as satiety due to the protein. Codfish is also lower in calories when compared to other types of fish, so it's highly considered a great food!

- **Eggs:** these are probably the best things you can eat in the morning for breakfast. High in protein, eggs will keep you going without snacks all morning. They are also very healthy and despite containing high levels of good cholesterol, they will not raise your bad cholesterol levels because they are not high in saturated fats.

- **Lentils:** one of the most popular sources of protein for vegetarians, lentils provide massive boosts of both protein and fiber to those who eat them. These two properties are key to losing weight and feeling full.

- **Prunes ("dried plums" in some countries):** I know a lot of people aren't fans of prunes, however, their health benefits are amazing! Prunes contain huge amounts of fiber, in particular, soluble fiber, which will not only keep your regular but also fill you up for hours!

- **Greens (any kind of leafy green vegetables):** as long as it's green and leafy, it's great for you! Quite simply, greens are so low in calories and also high in water content that they don't just fill you up but you can eat so much of them without having to worry about calories.

- **Peanut butter:** studies have shown that peanut butter is *very* healthy for you, providing it doesn't have added sugar or is processed (look for the all-natural peanut button in stores). Peanut butter does not raise cholesterol, and they have also been shown in studies to help with weight loss.

- **Pistachios:** compared to snacks like chips or pretzels, pistachios are much healthier. Studies have shown that they can reduce bad cholesterol when consumed in proper serving sizes (demonstrated later in this book).

- **Raisins:** yet another wonder food, raisins help to reduce hunger, which means less calories going into your body throughout the day! They also provide your body with antioxidants that support heart health.

- **Rye:** compared to other whole grains such as wheat, rye has many more positive benefits for your body. Shown to reduce your hunger for hours after eating it, rye will also help your body to cleanse itself due to the high fiber content.

- **Tofu:** many studies have shown that tofu, when compared to meats like chicken, not only keeps you feeling fuller for longer, but also supports blood pressure and cholesterol levels.

- **Whey protein:** often found in protein shakes and bars, whey protein is extracted from diary and has massive amounts of protein. It will reduce your caloric intake, keep you feeling very full, and reduce your appetite for hours!

Phase 1 Recipes

Super Almond Crackers

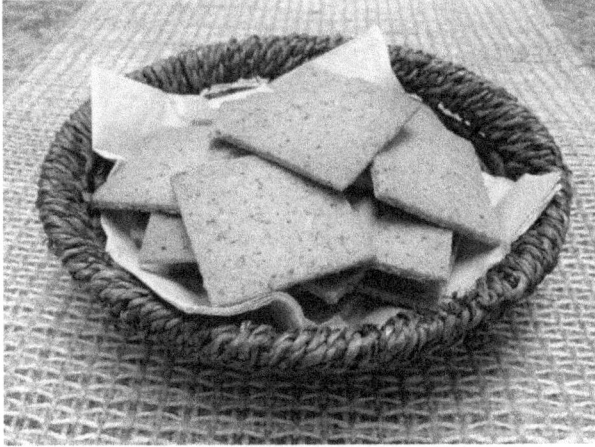

Ingredients

- 1 egg white
- 1 teaspoon of salt
- 1 cup of almond flour

Method

1. Firstly, combine and mix together the egg white, salt and almond flour until it turns into a paste texture.

2. Get your hands on a cookie sheet and some parchment paper. If you don't use the parchment paper you might run the risk of cracking your crackers once they're made.

3. Place the dough that you have made on the cookie sheet and make sure that you can roll it out thin (use a rolling pin if you need it).

4. Using a knife cut the dough into pieces that will later turn into your crackers.

5. Bake in the oven for about 10-15 minutes until they go crispy. Approximately 325 degrees Fahrenheit is perfect in terms of temperature.

6. Keep checking every few minutes to make sure you pull them out right when they're crispy. ENJOY!

Spicy Garlic Spinach & Kale

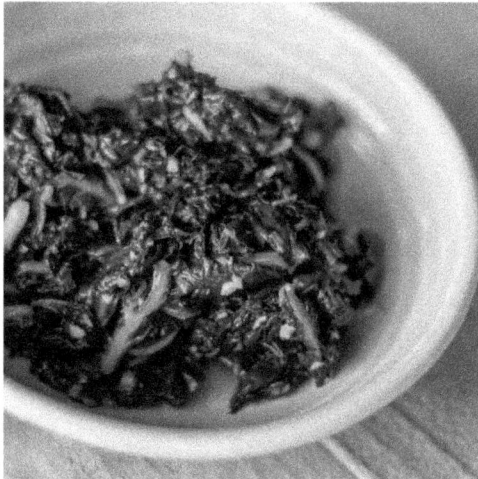

Ingredients

- 2 packs of baby spinach
- 4 kale leaves (despond them – remove stems)
- 1 teaspoon of garlic that is minced
- 2 teaspoons of light olive oil (regular olive oil works too)
- Red pepper flakes
- Sea salt and pepper (for additional taste and flavor if desired)

Method

1. Cut your kale into pieces that are about 1 inch in size.

2. Put both the olive oil and garlic into a pan (at medium heat) and continue to stir for a few minutes – make sure you don't burn the garlic!

3. Once it begins sizzling, you can add in the kale. Sauté until the oil is evenly dispersed.

4. Add in baby spinach and also sauté. Add in some red pepper flakes, and finally add some salt and pepper to taste.

5. Make sure that you don't burn the baby spinach or kale when adding them in. Remove from heat and serve. ENJOY!

Peanut Butter & Plums

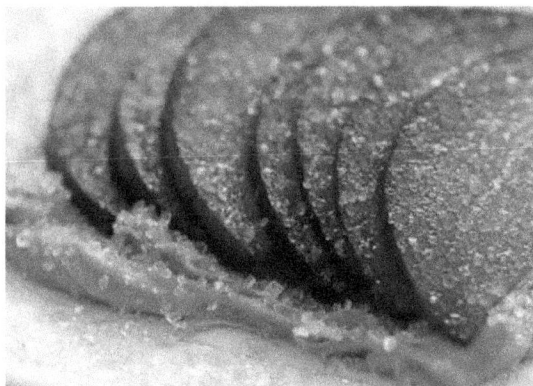

Ingredients

- 1 tablespoon of peanut butter
- 2 rye crackers
- 5 dried plums

Method

1. Spread the peanut butter on both the crackers. Serve with the dried plums.

2. If you wish, you can slice the dried plums and place them on top of the peanut butter for a mix of flavor. ENJOY!

Greenie Smoothie

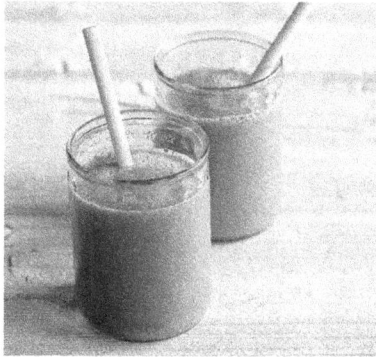

Ingredients

- 1 serve of Greek yogurt
- 1 Granny Smith apple with the skin on, sliced
- ¼ cup of spinach
- ¼ cup of whey protein powder
- 2 tablespoons of water
- 2 teaspoons of coconut oil

Method

1. Get your blender out. Toss in your yogurt, the slices of apple, the spinach, the protein powder and the water. Blend until it's smooth.

2. Add in the coconut oil and some ice. Blend once again until a consistency you are happy with. ENJOY!

Phase 2 Recipes

Fat Burn Granola

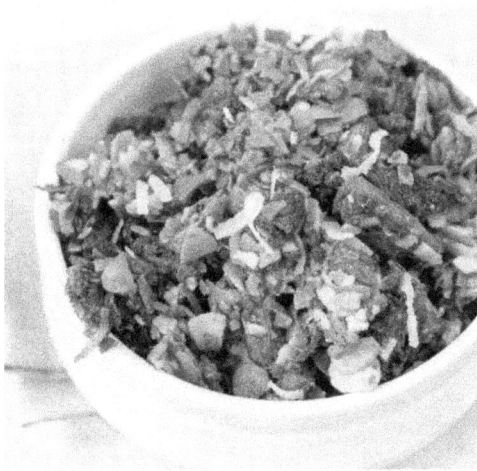

Ingredients

- 1 cup (approx. 227g) of slivered almonds
- 1 cup (approx. 227g) of cashews
- 3 cups of rolled oats
- ¾ cup of sweet coconut that is shredded
- ¼ cup of oil (preferably vegetable oil)
- ¼ cup of dark brown sugar with additional 2 tablespoons of dark brown sugar in case
- ¼ cup of maple syrup with additional 2 tablespoons of maple syrup
- ¾ teaspoon of salt
- 1 cup (approx. 227g) of raisins

Method

1. Before you begin, preheat your oven to 350 degrees Fahrenheit.

2. Get out two bowls, and put the coconut, oats, brown sugar and nuts in one bowl.

3. In the other bowl put your oil, maple syrup and salt.

4. Mix these bowls individually, and then combine together and pour all of it onto two sheet pans.

5. Leave it cooking for an hour; however, every 10-20 minutes try to stir so it achieves an even color and texture all over. Once done, take it out of the oven and keep it in a large bowl, adding raisins. ENJOY!

Spiced Omelet

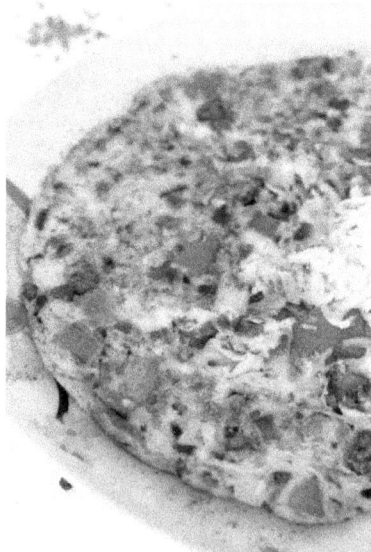

Ingredients

- 1 egg
- ¼ teaspoons of minced garlic
- 1 tablespoon of chopped cilantro
- 1 cup of spinach
- ½ cup of frozen, thawed corn
- ¼ sliced avocado
- 1 apple, skin on

Method

1. Whisk the egg together with both the minced garlic and the chopped cilantro.

2. Cook the above with the spinach and corn in a pan. Remove and serve on plate. Top with the sliced avocado. Serve with the apple. ENJOY!

Salad – Chicken & Corn

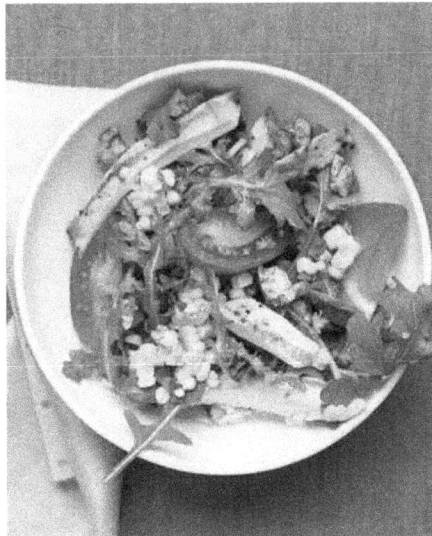

Ingredients

- 1 tablespoon of extra-virgin olive oil
- ½ tablespoon of balsamic vinegar
- ½ teaspoon of minced garlic
- 1 tablespoon of chopped cilantro
- 3 ounces of diced, boneless, cooked, skinless breast chicken
- ½ cup of frozen, thawed corn
- 1 cup of green leafy vegetables (of your choice)

Method

1. Cook the chicken on a pan. Toss in the corn and let it warm up. Remove and place in a bowl.

2. Add in the olive oil, vinegar, minced garlic, and cilantro and stir lightly. Serve with leafy greens. ENJOY!

Carrots & Hummus Combo

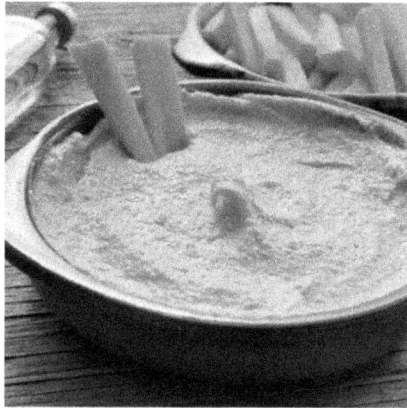

Ingredients

- ½ cup of chickpeas
- 2 teaspoons of extra-virgin olive oil

- ½ teaspoon of minced garlic
- 1 tablespoon of lemon juice
- 1 cup of raw baby carrots
- 2 rye crisps

Method

1. In a blender, purée the chickpeas, oil, minced garlic and lemon juice.

2. Serve the resulting hummus with the carrots and 2 rye crisps. Enjoy together!

Lemon Peppered Chicken Pasta

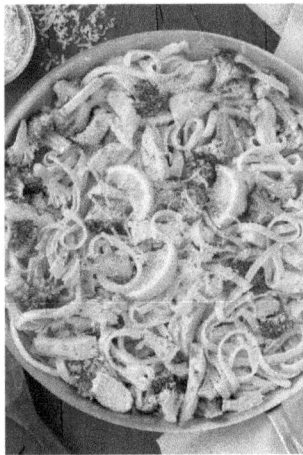

Ingredients

- ½ cup of grape tomatoes
- 1 tablespoon of extra-virgin olive oil
- ½ teaspoon of minced garlic
- ½ cup of cooked whole-grain rye pasta
- 1 cup of fresh spinach

- ½ tablespoon of lemon juice
- ¼ teaspoon of black pepper
- 3 ounces of diced, cooked, boneless, skinless chicken breast

Method

1. In a pan, sauté the grape tomatoes in the olive oil, along with the minced garlic.

2. Leave in the pan until the tomatoes are slightly tender. Remove and toss together with the cooked rye pasta.

3. Add in the spinach, lemon juice, black pepper, and cooked chicken. Stir all together. ENJOY!

Phase 3 Recipes

Protein-Packed Dijon Steak

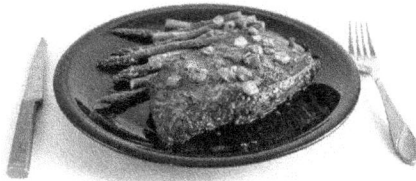

This recipe serves six people and it's INCREDIBLY simple!

Ingredients

- 1 tablespoon of honey
- 1 tablespoon of garlic salt
- 1 tablespoon of black and red pepper blend
- ½ a cup of Dijon mustard
- 1 and a ½ pounds of flank steak or boneless beef sirloin

Method

1. Take all the above ingredients, except the steak, and put it into a bowl. Mix well it well.

2. Take your steak out and spread the bowl of ingredients on both sides of your steak. Let it sit for about 5-10 minutes so the meat can absorb some of the flavor.

3. Grill your steaks over medium to high heat for about 6-10 minutes per side (depending on how well you like your steaks done). ENJOY!

Amazing Avocado Shrimp Salad

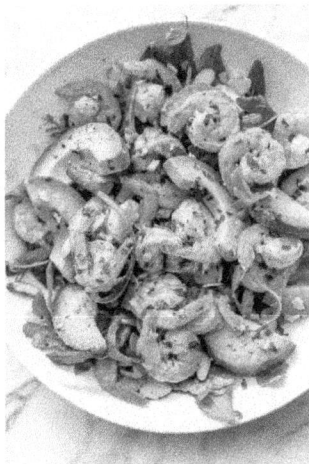

Ingredients

*   2 avocados, avoid cutting them too small, rather keep them in larger pieces
*   2 tablespoons of diced red onions
*   2lbs of steamed shrimp (boiled shrimp works fine too); peel and devein the shrimp too

Ingredients for the dressing

- ¼ cup of red wine vinegar
- ½ a teaspoon of garlic powder
- ¼ cup of extra virgin olive oil
- 1 teaspoon of Dijon mustard
- 1 teaspoon of chopped parsley
- Salt and pepper (only require for flavor if required)

Method

1. Get a large bowl and combine the shrimp, avocado and onion together, mixing well.

2. Take out a cup (if you have a double-cup this would be perfect), and combine all the above ingredients *only* for the dressing together. Mix these ingredients together very well (whisk if need be).

3. Once the dressing is ready, apply to the avocado shrimp salad and leave any remaining as a side. ENJOY!

Raspberry Butter Toast

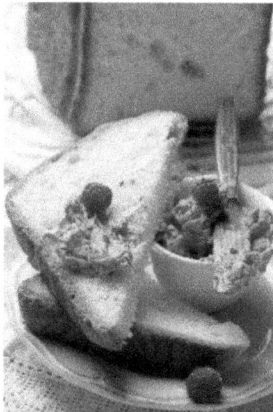

Ingredients

- 1 cup of raspberries
- ½ teaspoon of cinnamon
- 1 slice of whole-grain rye bread
- 1 cup of skim milk
- 1 tablespoon of peanut butter

Method

1. Mash the raspberries in a bowl. Once they have turned into a somewhat paste-like texture, add a sprinkle of cinnamon.

2. Toast the slice of bread. Spread the raspberry jam you have made, and top up with the peanut butter. If you wish, you can serve with a cup of skim milk. ENJOY!

Banana Butter Toast with Yogurt

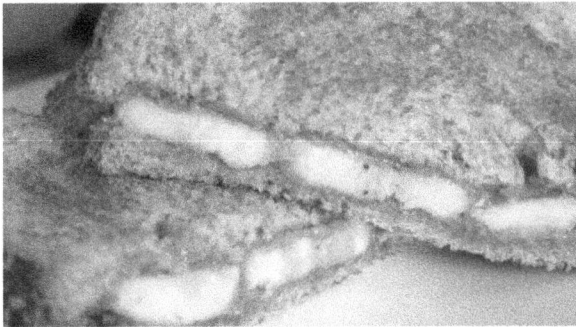

Ingredients

- 1 tablespoon of peanut butter
- 1 slice of whole-grain rye bread
- ½ cup of sliced up banana
- 1 serving of low fat/non-fat Greek yogurt

Method

1. Toast your bread. Spread the peanut butter on your bread.

2. Top the bread with your sliced bananas. Serve with a side of yogurt. ENJOY!

Chicken & Wild Rice Lettuce Wraps

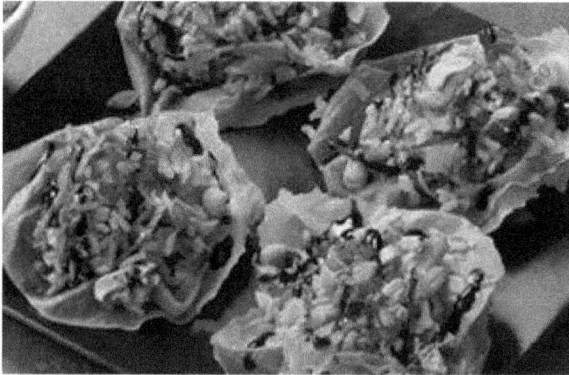

Ingredients

- 3 ounces of chicken (boneless, skinless, diced)
- 1 tablespoon of extra-virgin olive oil
- ½ teaspoon of minced garlic and salt-free Italian herb seasoning
- 2 large romaine lettuce leaves
- 2 tablespoons of wild rice
- ¼ cup minced red onion
- ½ cup chopped grape tomatoes

Method

1. Cook your chicken first; lightly fry on a pan with the extra virgin olive oil.

2. Add in the minced garlic and salt-free Italian herb seasoning. Remove and put in a bowl.

3. Fill the lettuce leaves with cooked and chilled wild rice. Add in the red onion and grape tomatoes. Wrap the leaves and serve with the chicken. ENJOY!

Napa Valley Snack

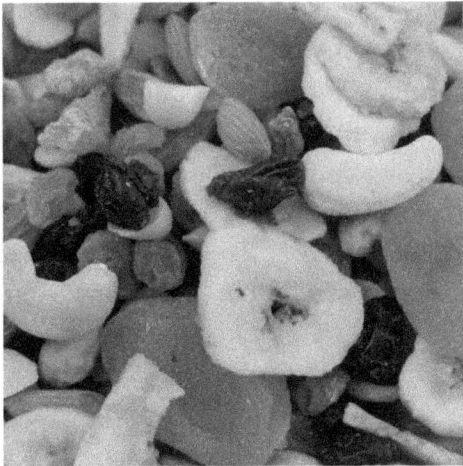

Ingredients

- 2 rye crisps
- 1 mini-round of cheese
- 1 pear with the skin
- 2 tablespoons of walnuts

Method

1. Spread the cheese on the rye crisps.

2. Serve with the pear. Also serve with the walnuts. Makes for a great snack during the day. ENJOY!

Full Body Transformation – Weight Loss System

This section will teach you the full weight loss system. If you're a beginner, I recommend that you go through the Kick Starter Program first, then follow into this after Day 31. For those who feel they are intermediate or advanced, and have been losing weight already or live a somewhat healthy life and just need to lose less than 20lbs, then you can go straight into this section.

You will get a comprehensive understanding of the theory behind weight loss, understanding what makes food healthy and what makes food unhealthy. You will get a massive list of recipes too! Additionally, I have included some of the most effective workouts to burn fat and improve fitness. They are scientifically proven from case studies and also focused on particular areas of the body.

Module 1

How It Works

This weight loss system is basically a weight loss plan that anyone who desires to have a full body transformation can follow! This is no exaggeration: the action-packed procedures detailed in this book are effective and easy to carry out. The plan is broken up into some actionable steps (in each module) that would necessitate maximum body transformation.

Fundamentals of good food

Here, you will learn about the fundamentals of good food. There are six classes of food, namely carbohydrates, proteins, fat, minerals, water and vitamins. The first three classes are referred to as macronutrients, because human body needs them in substantial amounts for metabolic processes. You will discover the inherent magic in these classes of food, and how they can be instrumental in loosening up the fat in your body within a very short period of time.

Recipes for effective weight-loss

From module **three** to **six**, you will be exposed to some fat-burning recipes for breakfasts, lunches, dinners and snacks. Each chapter has five sample recipes you can prepare and consume to shed appreciable amount of weight! The good thing about these recipes is that they could be localized: that is, you can find the active ingredients for the recipes in your geographic location or utilize some other local ingredients that offer similar properties.

Fundamentals of good workouts

As reflected in this book, a great weight-loss system must combine both the dietary requirements with excellent workouts that are capable of producing believable outcomes. Two modules are entirely dedicated to two different types of workouts for anyone who is truly serious about losing weight– cardio and resistance training. These two ground-breaking exercises/workouts have been known to be quite effective and harmless.

Final tips for success

Here is where you will find all the necessary steps put together in the form of a checklist. You can view it as a list or summary of essential steps that must be taken in order to effectively lose your weight!

The Naked Truth

A lot of diet books out there leave you feeling bad about yourself, especially if you slip up once in a while. This is not one of those books. The aim of this book is to help you to feel good about yourself. All I am going to ask you to do is to commit to yourself and this simple weight loss system and I promise that you will come out of it with renewed self-confidence.

Let's Dive Right in

To start off with, you are going to get to grips with the body you have – Yippee, your first chance to get naked! The first step is to have a good look at your body in the mirror. When last did you actually do that? I started doing some research and guess what? Everyone has some part of themselves that they are insecure about. In fact, Glamour Magazine polled its readers and found that 97% think negative thoughts about their bodies EVERY day.

A friend of mine, one of the slimmest people I know, is constantly on a diet. She insists that she needs to lose 10lbs. No one except her can see where this mysterious extra 10lbs is, but she controls what she eats with an iron fist. Then, every now and again she cannot take it anymore and she binges. She ends up feeling disgusted with herself and then once again goes into "diet" mode.

Despite being so slim, she has a really bad body image and, until she works on that, she is always going to feel unattractive. And that is what I am going to teach you about in this book – accepting your own body for what it is, as it is now. So, let's get back to that mirror, shall we? What do you hate about your body? What do you love about it? Make notes. Now comes the tough part – for every negative you put down, you need to have at least one positive. You don't get to put your clothes back on until you've completed this exercise, so start looking.

When I did this exercise for the first time, I did battle to balance the list. Then I started to think about it for a bit – my body is actually an amazing machine. What we tend to forget is that our bodies are incredible – no matter what shape they are. There is always something to love. Now that you have your list, it is time to get down to the basics of the program.

Understanding the System

This program works because it encourages you to think differently about your body from the outset. In the next chapter, I will explain why this is so important to your success. I will then move on to discuss the principles of healthy eating and give you the 7-Day Food Plan. I will then give tips on how to really amp up the results before moving on to dealing with specific areas of the body.

The last part of the program deals with grooming and general trouble shooting. On completion of the program, you will look better and, more importantly, feel better. The principles that you learn here can be incorporated into your everyday life after you have finished the program. This is not a weight loss plan, it is a lifestyle plan and will help you feel great inside and out.

To the Start Line Please

To start off with, let's set some goals. What is it that you would like to get out of this program? Set yourself some goals – maybe you want to trim your waistline a little, maybe you want to lose a whole lot of weight or perhaps you just want to feel healthier. Whatever your goal, set it down in writing.

Now consider what it is going to take for you to achieve that goal and set up a realistic timeframe. If you do have a lot of weight to lose, setting it out in written format can be a bit daunting. Break it down into mini-goals. Setting yourself a target of losing 10lbs is a lot less daunting than setting a target of 100lbs.

A further advantage of setting up mini-goals is that achieving them is motivation in itself.

Take a Photo, It Lasts Longer

Now you need to take a "Before" picture of yourself. This will provide you with visual evidence of exactly how far you have come. Right now it's Ready, Steady Go!

It Starts in Your Head

Pick up any just about any magazine and you are bombarded with pictures of gorgeous people – perfect skin and perfect bodies. There is no denying it; we are a very image-conscious society. We are told that this is the way we were meant to look. What we are not told is how much work went into getting those picture-perfect results.

What if I were to tell you that with a few tweaks, you too could grace the pages of a fashion magazine? All it takes to look that perfect is a great makeup artist and hairstylist, great photo-imaging software and a few clicks of the mouse. Photo-editing software is so advanced now that it is possible to completely change the look of the original photo.

Just as an example, I edited one of my brother's wedding photos. I not only removed two people from the photo completely but I even changed the beach in the background. And I am an amateur. Imagine what the professionals can do. Have you ever seen a picture of Kate Moss without makeup on, for example? You probably wouldn't recognize her if you walked past her in the street. Models are slim and trim but at least 40% of them acknowledge that they have some form of eating disorder.

Magazine editors know that we want to see pictures of beautiful people and they oblige with an image of perfection that is not only false but that is not representative of the average person out there. The message we get all around us is clear – you need to aim to be perfect all the time if you want to be successful. No wonder so many people have a negative body image.

Time to Turn It Around

Take a look at the list you made in the chapter before and look at the negative comments you made about yourself. There is a good chance that you think these things quite often. I'll bet that you found it pretty easy to list the negatives and a lot harder to list the positives. Most people can rattle off a list of things that they hate about their bodies without giving it too much thought.

The problem is that the more we think a thought, the more we believe it. It gets engrained into our psyche and our minds accept this as fact. As Henry Ford said, "Whether you think you can, or you think you can't, you're right." This is where the real danger of negative thinking comes in. We start to create our own reality based on these thoughts – whether they are realistic or not.

The mind then starts looking for more evidence to back up these thoughts and prove that they are true – you feel worse about yourself and the whole cycle starts up again. With this mindset, it is very difficult to make positive changes to the way that you look. You need to break the cycle and learn how to accept your body for what it is now. That means switching off the negative talk and changing the message that you are sending to your body.

The payoffs in doing this are quite astounding – remember that whatever your mind focuses on becomes a part of your reality. Keep sending positive thoughts to your brain and you will find that it starts to look for evidence to support this new way of thinking. You will start to feel happier in yourself and you will find that it will be easier to drop extra weight and to stick to a healthy eating plan and exercise schedule.

How to Change your Mindset

Changing your mindset is going to take a bit of work but will be easier than you think.

Get as Much Information as Possible

Think about something that you know little to nothing about. In my case, I'll say playing field hockey. I believe that hockey is a dangerous sport. I have never played hockey in my life because of this belief. A woman that I once worked with loved hockey and played twice a week – she never had so much as a bruised shin in the three years that I worked with her.

I still won't be joining a hockey team any time soon but that is more because I am not a fan of sport rather than because I am afraid of getting hurt. I know now that field hockey is not as dangerous as I first believed because I am better educated about it. I understand it better so I am able to make an informed decision. Being properly informed is vital when it comes to changing your mindset. Get rid of all that misinformation that you have about weight loss and fitness and get to grips with the facts. You'll find that you are a lot more confident when you know what you are talking about.

Be Mindful of your Thoughts

Start to monitor your thoughts – your inner critic can be quite ruthless at times and sometimes you need to tell it to shut up. If you catch yourself thinking something negative about your body, actively turn that thought into a positive one.

Ask yourself the following:

- **Is this absolutely true?** "I'll never lose weight" was one of my favorite personal mantras. There was no truth in that statement because I had proven that I was capable of losing weight previously.

- **Would I say this to my best friend?** If your best friend said to you that they would never lose weight, what would you tell them? You would try to talk them round, wouldn't you? You are probably meaner to yourself than you would be to someone you dislike. Does that make any sense at all?

- **Am I comparing myself to someone else?** If so, stop it at once. Everyone is different and everyone has problems of their own.

- **Will thinking this help me feel good about myself?** If not, it really is not a worthwhile thought – you deserve to feel good about yourself, everyone does.

Change "Should" to "Could"

Every time you start to say, "I should..." see what happens if you change that to "I could ...." You will be amazed at what a difference this can make. "Should" puts more pressure on you and, in your mind, it takes the choice away from you. How do you usually feel about things that you should do? For example, "I should eat more vegetables."

If you change that phrase around to, "I could eat more vegetables" and it puts the power back in your hands – you could make the choice to eat more vegetables or you could make the choice not to – it is your decision.

Fake it until you make it

This is a lesson that I learned from Louise Hay – every day you need to stand in front of the mirror and say, "I love you" to your reflection. I have to admit, that I did feel quite silly about doing this the first few times but once I got into the habit of doing this it became a lot easier.

Step up to your mirror every day with a big smile on your face and say, "I love you." Add at least five things that you like about your body. If it helps, write little notes for yourself and put them on the mirror. Leave little notes for yourself around the house so that you come upon them randomly. Over time this positive reinforcement will start to sink in and you will develop a healthier body image.

Watch Your Body Language

Projecting an aura of confidence is half the battle won. Look at someone that you admire for their confidence – how do they walk? How do they carry themselves? Human beings are very quick to pick up on non-verbal cues and, if your body language is screaming that you want to slip by unnoticed, people are not going to take much notice of you. You must not hide behind your fat here either – it is easier to say that people just aren't attracted to you because of your weight but the truth is that it is a lot more complicated than that.

It depends on the vibes that you send out – if you do not feel that you are worth getting to know, why should other people? I can personally vouch for that. I used to believe that I had no control over what others thought about me. I knew that I was overweight and unattractive and that no man would ever love me because of this. I lost 10 years of my life because of this – I believed that I was unlovable and so I put out that vibe.

One of my brother's friends got me to turn this around. She was about the same weight as me and yet, when she went out, she had guys hitting on her every time. The big difference was that she exuded confidence – she liked herself for who she was and carried herself accordingly.

58

Dress for Success

You need at least one outfit that makes you look and feel great now, at the size you are now. Read up on dressing to suit your body shape and to create a slimmer, more streamlined effect. Go through the clothes in your wardrobe – either get rid of anything that is shapeless or alter them so that they fit better. Contrary to popular belief, fitted clothing is more slimming than baggy clothing.

Module 2

The ONE Thing That Will Determine Your Success

Eating the right food is essential to getting your perfect bikini as quickly as possible. This module outlines the main types of foods that this system offers.

The Calorie Factor

Calories are effectively very simple. We eat a lot of food and drink, all full of calories, every day. When we eat more than we burn off, or don't move enough to use up the calories then we put on weight. In order to reverse that and lose weight, we need to eat less and move more, sure, but we need to do it in the right way, especially if we want a body that is fit to show off in a bikini at the end of it. Everything we eat or drink has some calorific value, apart from water, which we will look at shortly.

Food and drink that we take for granted as part of everyday normal meals such as potatoes, wine, red meat and cheese is typically high in calories, so we need to cut it right down if we want to shed the pounds, or in the case of alcohol, cut it out completely for a while. An average man needs around 2500 calories a day to maintain his weight. For an average woman, that figure is around 2000 calories a day. Some plans recommend that you reduce just 500 calories per day. You will lose weight, but you can drop pounds faster and in just as healthy a manner with this diet, which takes you closer to 1000 calories per day. It is not recommended that anyone drop below 1000 calories per day when trying to lose weight. But there is no calorie-counting necessary with this plan, just choose the meals you want from the selection. Losing weight is well worth the effort and not just for looks. Being overweight or obese causes an increased risk of type 2 diabetes, heart disease, stroke and some cancers. Lose a few pounds and you drastically reduce the health risks.

Fat Facts

Everybody some fat to function properly. But compare it to other macronutrients:

Protein: 1 gram = 4 calories
Carbohydrates: 1 gram = 4 calories
Alcohol: 1 gram = 7 calories
Fat: 1 gram = 9 calories

Eat too much fat and, at 9 calories per gram, it will obviously be fattening. However, not all fats stack up the same nutritionally and some fats are better for you than others. Polyunsaturated fats, which come from plants, are best, saturated animal fats should be minimized and trans fats from processed foods should be avoided altogether. Other good fats come from fish. Salmon and tuna are high in protein, and contain essential omega-3 fatty acids. These have been shown to regulate a hormone called leptin, which is involved in enabling an increased caloric burn.

The Carbs Quandary

Starchy carbohydrates – potatoes, rice, pasta, bread and so on - act just like sugar in the body, spiking the blood and causing a surge of insulin, which commands the body to hold onto the calories as fat.

In this diet, the starchy carbs are strictly limited. However, if you cut them out completely, then eat them later you can find that you simply put weight straight back on.

We want your weight loss to be both highly effective and lasting, so we encourage you to enjoy light amount of carbs as part of this diet. You will find that this helps to curb your hunger and also keeps your metabolism burning brightly.

Drinking Well

Throughout this plan you will:

- Avoid alcohol. Liquor is bad for dieting all round, as it is very high in calories and it saps your energy, acts as a depressant and slows your metabolism. Plus, you should never exercise when you have been drinking!

- Not drink regular coffee or tea at all as these are packed with the stimulant caffeine. Herbal infusions and rooibos/red bush tea are fine.

- Avoid all energy drinks as they are simply packed with added sugar, often labeled under other names like 'glucose' and so on.

- Above all drink lots of water, 6-8 glasses per day. Your metabolism, digestive system, whole body and brain work at their best when properly hydrated – this is a major key to weight loss so keep topping up your glass with the clear stuff.

If you feel like sharing the love and helping other readers decide if this is the right book for them, please take a few seconds to leave a short review on Amazon.com.

The Theory of Good Food

You are what you eat! Whilst I don't want to "be" a piece of lettuce, I'm also not fond of the idea of looking like a donut. Thing of your body in the same way as you would a precise German engineered car – if you put the wrong fuel in it, it won't perform as it should and will eventually break down. It's the same with your body – eating the wrong foods will cause problems in the long run. Except in our case, there are very few replacement parts.

Good Wholesome Food

You need to rethink what you are eating – the aim should be to eat food that is as close to natural as possible. The more a food is processed, the less nutritious it becomes – you could be eating 6 meals a day and still not be getting the nutrients that you need.

Here are the basic guidelines for good eating habits:

Ditch the Sugar

And I don't mean just the sugar that you add to your tea or coffee, I mean all the hidden sugars as well. It is estimated that the average American eats about 156 pounds of sugar a year. Only 29% of that total is in the form of sucrose – your normal sugar. The rest is in the form of the sugar added to your food and beverages.

Take a walk around your local grocery store and have a look at the ingredients of some of the foods on the shelves. Look for words like "sucrose" and "high fructose corn syrup". Check how near the top of the list of ingredients these sugars are. Ingredients are labeled in the order of the proportion contained within the food – the higher they appear on the list, the higher the proportion of that ingredient in the food itself. You will be shocked to find how many items contain sugar and, in most cases, it will be in the top five ingredients of the product.

Sugar is added to just about everything these days – it is a cheap and easy way to enhance the flavor of foods. Even the so-called healthy options often contain a lot of sugar. Your flavored waters, for example, can contain almost as much sugar as a normal soda. Take a look at the healthy cereals that you are feeding your kids. If sugar is not top of the list, it is probably pretty close. Many of the so-called healthy, low fat foods contain a lot of sugar – fat helps to give the food its satisfying flavor. Without fat, the food tastes quite bland so the manufacturers add a lot of sugar to improve the flavor.

Starting today, you need to clear out the sugar from your diet. Check the ingredients of everything that you buy – if sugar is in the top five ingredients; put it back on the shelf. We have heard a lot over the years about the dangers of fat. Sugar is just as dangerous if we consume too much. The problem is that sugar contains a both fructose and glucose. Your whole body is able to use the glucose. The fructose, on the other hand, can only be used by the liver. In the liver it is converted to glycogen for use as energy.

There is only so much fructose that the liver can metabolize – the rest is converted to fat. Some of this fat gets stored in the liver and this can cause fatty liver syndrome – a harmful and potentially deadly condition. That is not the worst of it though - sugar is easily absorbed into the blood stream – your blood sugar levels spike and the body goes into overdrive to rebalance them. It does this by flooding the body with insulin. If this happens once in a while, it is not such a big issue. If it happens on a repeated basis, however, the body starts to build up a resistance to the insulin and it becomes less and less effective. In time, the cells in the pancreas become damaged and you develop adult onset diabetes.

Insulin is also responsible for getting the body to store fat instead of using it. The more insulin in the blood stream, the more your body will hold onto its fat. This also causes weight gain. Added sugar can also cause changes in your blood lipid profile, most importantly raising the levels of triglycerides. The triglycerides interfere with the action of Leptin – one of the hormones that tell the brain to stop eating and to burn more energy. Our bodies become resistant to Leptin and the brain interprets this as a sign that more food is needed.

And last but not least, sugar is addictive. Confirming what choc-aholics have long suspected, sugar does make you feel good. It acts on the dopamine center in the brain so we feel pleasure when eating sugar. Over time, your body develops a physical addiction to sugar. Added sugar has no significant nutritional value either. There is no good reason to add it to your daily diet. Cut it out of your diet today.

Bye Bye Processed Foods

Processed foods contain very little in terms of nutritional value. For the most part, they contain large quantities of unhealthy trans-fats, little or no fiber, lots of sugar and a whole range of chemical additives. The rule of 5 applies here too – if a product has 5 or more ingredients, it has no business being in your shopping cart.

Add in Protein

Protein is needed by every part of our body and most especially by our muscles. It is used for repair and the production of energy. If you do not get enough protein in your diet, you will feel lethargic and your body will not recover as quickly after exercise. It contains essential amino acids that the body needs to build and repair muscle tissue. Protein helps to slow down the absorption of sugar into the blood and helps you to feel fuller for longer. To get the best effects, you need to add in a portion of high-quality protein with every meal and snack. This may sound like a lot at first but it really is not.

Here are some easy ways to gauge how much one serving of protein is for you:

- A matchbox size of cheese. (Alternatively, cut wafer thin slices of cheese using a potato peeler; nine of these slices will count as one serving.)
- A piece of meat that is as big as your palm and the same thickness as your hand
- 1 small tub of natural yoghurt
- A handful of nuts or seeds
- 1 egg – yolk and all
- A piece of salmon about the size of a deck of cards

Finding ways to add in extra protein is especially important if you want to look better naked. Protein helps your body to build more muscle. Muscle, in turn, burns more energy when at rest than fat does. Changing the muscle to fat ratio in your body can help to boost your weight loss efforts significantly.

All You Need is Love, and Fiber

Fiber is another essential element when it comes to losing weight. You need both soluble and insoluble fibers. Soluble fibers are necessary in order to help feed the beneficial bacteria in your gut. It is these bacteria that are an essential part of ensuring that your digestive system is healthy and as efficient as it should be.

Soluble fibers help to reduce the rate at which sugar is absorbed into your blood stream. They thus help to normalize blood sugar levels and prevent dangerous drops in energy. Insoluble fiber helps to make you feel fuller with less food – the more fiber there is in an item of food, the more filling it is. It also helps to move things along in the intestinal tract. You can get plenty of fiber from fruits and vegetables.

Add in Some Fruit and Veggies

Around about half of your plate should be covered in low-carb veggies such as lettuce, tomatoes, etc. and add in a serving of low G.I. fruits at snack time. You should get about 5-9 servings of fruit and veggies a day. Fruits are great but do contain a lot of natural sugars so it is best to stick to the lower G.I. varieties such as apples and berries. If you are trying to lose weight, it is better to avoid fruits with high sugar content such as grapes. If, however, you are really craving something sweet, it is better to reach for a piece of fruit than for a candy bar.

Where possible, eat the skin of the fruit or vegetable as well as this is where the highest concentration of fiber is. You should also eat the whole fruit or vegetable – whilst a lot has been said on the benefits of juicing, the truth is that juicing removes most of the fiber so it will not keep you feeling full throughout the day. Fruit juices, especially store-bought ones, are best avoided altogether as they very often have a lot of added sugar. Try to get the very freshest produce that you can manage – even grow your own if you can. The fresher the produce, the better it tastes. Stick to food that is in season and try to source it at your local farmer's market. If you cannot get fresh, frozen is the next best thing. Avoid canned fruit and veggies altogether. You should aim for variety as well in order to get the best nutrient value.

Add in a Portion of Fat

I know that over the years we have all been told how bad fat is for us. The latest research is now showing that sugar is actually a lot more fattening than fat is. Experts now believe that at least 35% of your daily calories should come from fat. The trick is to eat the right kinds of fats. Your body needs healthy fats in order to operate properly. If it does not get enough, it will hang onto the fat stores that it already has.

The key here is the word healthy. You need to cut out trans-fats completely – trans-fats are created when the fat is subjected to high heats and the chemical bonds within the fats are changed. Tans-fats have been linked to higher levels of inflammation and provide very little nutrition for your body. You should ensure that the majority of your fats are either mono-unsaturated fats or saturated fats. The advantage of eating more fat is that the food tastes better. Cook your food using olive oil or coconut oil – both are resistant to high temperatures and their structure remains healthy. Monounsaturated fats are essential if you are trying to get a flat belly and you should have one serving at every meal.

Again, this is not as much as it may seem to be at first:

- 10 large olives
- 2 tablespoons of nuts
- 1 tablespoon of olive oil
- Half an avocado
- A serving of salmon

Fats also help to slow the absorption of sugar into the blood and are high on the satiety index – they help you feel fuller for longer. They also help to make your food taste great. Steak and baked potato served with butter with a side salad makes for a very satisfying and tasty meal – and can be eaten with this diet.

Tips to Boost your Metabolism

- Calorie counting is not as important as it was once thought to be. By adding protein and a serving of fat to each meal, you are ensuring that your meals are more filling. You will find that you get full faster. Protein also takes a lot of energy for the body to process so just by eating more protein you will lose weight.

- Have at least 3 cups of green tea every day – doing this alone can boost metabolism by around 10%. Green tea helps to rev up the metabolism because of its caffeine content. Green tea is packed full of antioxidants and so helps to fight inflammation. This is great news for your skin. You need to drink it without milk for the best effects.

- Muscle is your friend when it comes to your metabolic rate. Muscle burns more calories than fat throughout the day.

- Drink enough water. If your body does not get enough water every day, your metabolic rate slows down in order to conserve it. You need to drink around about 8 – 10 glasses at the very least.

- Don't be afraid to add spice to your meals – hot peppers and chilies can fire up your taste buds and your metabolism.

- Exercise in and of itself will also boost the metabolism.

- Interval training keeps your body guessing and makes it harder for the body to get used to your physical fitness routine. If you keep doing the same workouts over and over again, your body becomes more efficient at them and so you will burn fewer calories. Switching this up helps improve overall efficiency.

A Simple Exercise to Boost Metabolism

Cardio combined with any of the strength training exercises will help you to boost your metabolism. This 30-minute walk-run-interval session (plus warm-up and cool-down) gives you maximum calorie burn in minimum time to help you work getting fit into your crazy schedule. Do it 3 times a week.

1. Walk briskly for 5 minutes to warm up.
2. Run at a moderate pace for 7 minutes, and then walk briskly for 3 minutes.
3. Run at a slightly faster pace for 3 minutes, and then walk briskly for 2 minutes.
4. Repeat steps 2 and 3.
5. Run at a slow pace for 3 minutes, and then walk for 2 minutes to cool down.

Daily Supplements to Consider

You do not need a whole lot of different supplements but a daily multi-vitamin is very important. One of the main reasons that the body causes you to crave things is that it is deficient in one nutrient or another. Whilst this diet will go a long way towards correcting a nutrient imbalance, it is still very difficult to get all the nutrients that you need from diet alone. You will need a good quality multi-vitamin supplement. Look for one with a balanced range of vitamins and minerals. This provides nutritional backup for you.

You may also need to take an Omega 3 supplement – Omega 3s are vital to health and vitality but most of us are deficient in them. Our bodies cannot produce them ourselves. Our bodies do not readily convert plant sources of Omega 3s. A fish oil supplement, or two-three servings of oily fish a week are what you need to get enough of this fatty acid. Cod liver oil is the best bet here – even if you are eating oily fish it is not guaranteed that you will get the right levels of Omega 3s. Even though salmon is an oily fish, there is a difference between farmed salmon and wild salmon and this can make a significant difference to their Omega 3 content.

Chromium is another supplement to consider, particularly if you feel that you may have developed insulin resistance. Chromium helps to balance blood sugar levels naturally. As far as vitamin supplements go, this is really all that you will need. When it comes to mega-doses of vitamins, you are, at best, wasting your money and, at worst, possibly poisoning your body.

Extra water-soluble vitamins such as Vitamin C will simply be flushed out of the body. Extra fat-soluble vitamins such as Vitamin E will be stored in the fat tissues and this could lead to toxic levels building up. If you are really under a lot of pressure, you could supplement your Vitamin B intake as well. There is some talk that Vitamin B makes you hungrier but this is really only true if you are really deficient in the nutrient and then the effect is only temporary anyway.

Another supplement to consider initially is a Milk Thistle supplement. This provides support for the liver and helps it to get rid of toxins that have built up in the system. It also helps to boost the metabolism of fat in the body. As with a lot of natural supplements, you should use this for a month and then give it a break for at least two weeks. Fiber is a very important part of your daily diet and, as such, you should consider a daily supplement in order to get the optimal doses. Take it in the morning for the best effect. Be sure to have a big glass of water with the supplement in order to get the best effects.

Spices to Add

Spices are essential in making food taste good but they can also have a very real impact on metabolism and blood sugar as well.

- Cayenne pepper helps to increase the metabolic rate and decrease levels of inflammation in your system. Use in daily cooking or take a half teaspoon in a little water with your breakfast in the morning. It does not taste good to take it this way but it is a good way to ensure that you get a full daily dose.

- Cinnamon is very effective at balancing blood sugar levels. Start with a half teaspoon a day – either sprinkle over food or add in when cooking. Cinnamon is so effective that people on medication to control diabetes or insulin resistance are advised to monitor their sugar levels carefully to ensure that the levels do not drop too low. Combined with a Chromium supplement, cinnamon is particularly potent.

- Turmeric is great at helping reduce inflammation in the system and supplementation with it has been shown promising results in line with the effects of some anti-inflammatory drugs. You can add it to your food but ideally you need a supplement that provides about 1000mg of Curcumin – the active ingredient in Turmeric a day.

Fundamentals of Food

According to food science, there are six classes of food, namely carbohydrates, proteins, fat, minerals, water and vitamins. The first three classes are called macronutrients, because they are mainly responsible for the series of daily metabolic activities going on in human body system. In the same way, vitamins, water and minerals are also integral parts of human metabolism.

Let's briefly consider the active components of these food classes:

- **Carbohydrates:** Carbohydrates are rich in dietary fibers and they include foods like breads, breakfast cereals, rice, pasta, noodles, potato, fruits, starchy vegetables, corn, dried beans and so on. Carbohydrates are generally low in saturated fat and energy (calories). They are essential constituents of any weight-loss dietary plan.

- **Proteins:** Your body can obtain proteins from both animal and plant sources, and they are mainly responsible for the growth and repair of cells in human body. You can get proteins from meat, chicken, eggs, nuts, dried beans and lentils, soy products, dairy products like milk, yoghurt and eggs.

- **Fat:** There are two distinct categories of fat—unsaturated and saturated fat. Unsaturated fat is very good for your body because they reduced the quantity of cholesterol in the blood and prevent cardiac or heart problems. You can get unsaturated fat by consuming food items like walnuts, cashew nuts, canola oil, soy products, flaxseed, soybean oil, safflower, and Brazil nuts. On the other hand, unsaturated fat is the chief cause of headache for people because it dangerously raises the amount of cholesterol in human blood and mostly instigate cardiac or heart problem. You can get saturated fat from foods like butter, ice-cream, dairy products, custard, cheese, fatty cuts of beef, pork, chicken, palm oil, coconut oil, cooking margarine, fatty snack foods, deep-fried foods, packaged cakes and biscuits, pastries and pies. Saturated fat is what makes people get fat indeed!

- **Water:** Human body is made up of 70 percent of water. This is why it advisable to drink a lot of it during hot weather or when you are exercising. It is imperative that you keep the water level in your body intact so that there wouldn't be any hitch in the water-aided metabolic activities going on in your body.

- **Minerals:** Your body needs some macronutrients to function properly. These nutrients include but are not limited to calcium, phosphorus, potassium, sulfur, chloride, iron, sodium, manganese and zinc. They are very useful in the development of cells in human body.

- **Vitamins:** Your body needs a little amount of vitamins, which are organic compounds required for human growth. You can get vitamins from foods and fruits, your body can also synthesize some vitamins, for instance, Vitamin K and D.

You may want to ask: how do these classes of food help people to lose weight? Don't people naturally get fat by eating the same classes of food? Dieticians and nutritionists explain that having a balanced diet—a practice of eating only the amount of food that your body needs to function properly—is the surest way to keep fat away.

People get fat when they start eating indiscriminately: some food is rich in fat, while others aren't. Eating good food in required quantities is the way to go if you are genuinely determined to shed pounds. Before you sit down to eat any kind of food, think about this: Will this food help me burn the fat in my body? Will it increase the rate of the metabolic processes going on in my body system? Will it reduce the level of cholesterol in my body? Research has shown that the six categories of foods outlined below are indeed the **six top fat-burning foods.**

- **Whole grains:** Consuming whole grains like brown rice and oatmeal help your body to burn fat twice faster than when you eat processed foods. Whole grains contain high percentage of fiber, and they are helpful for mopping up the extra fat in your body.

- **Lean meat:** Lean meat, a common source of protein to the body, is regarded as being thermogenic. That is, during digestion, your body can burn or break down 30 percent of the calories the meat contains. This high rate of combustion makes it impossible to leave chunk of fat in your body when consumed.

- **Low-fat dairy products:** The good thing about low-fat dairy products is that they contain minerals and vitamins, like calcium and vitamin D, which assist metabolism and cell growth in your body.

- **Green Tea:** A famous *American Journal of Clinical Nutrition* report states that drinking four cups of green tea a day will help you lose about 8 pound of weight in eight weeks. The tea reportedly contains EGCG, a compound that speeds up metabolic process in human body.

- **Lentils:** Lentils provide the iron required for metabolism to your body. Human body is composed of 20 percent of iron, and whenever there is a deficiency of this vital nutrient in human body, metabolic activities will be slow and inefficient.

- **Hot peppers:** Do you know how hot you usually feel when you eat hot peppers? It is due to capsaicin, a compound found in raw, dried, cooked and powdered pepper, which heats up your body and force some stubborn calories in your body to melt.

Though it is good knowing what kinds of benefits you can derive from different types of food, but what is very important is that you should only consume a small quantity of such foods. Over-eating is a gateway to putting on unnecessary fat that could make your life miserable.

The Ultimate 7-Day FAT-BLASTING Food Plan

Here is a sample meal plan for you so that you can see exactly what I was talking about throughout this module. The calorie content is not as important as getting the right nutrients so you can adjust this plan to suit yourself, as long as you are following the principles I have laid out. It is important to eat every 2-3 hours or so as this will help to rev up your metabolism for the whole day. This is also key when it comes to keeping your blood sugar at an even keel – you will have a steady flow of energy throughout the day and no nasty sugar crashes. That afternoon slump is not normal – it is a sign that you are not eating properly. The benefit of this plan is that you will not feel hungry and that the foods will help to boost your mood. Finally, of course, this meal plan alone will help you blast fat and lose anywhere between 2 to 15 pounds in JUST 7 days!

Disclaimer: for you to lose in the upper range of that claim above (around 15lbs), you need to follow the meal plan strictly, ensure you are drinking adequate water (at least a gallon a day, depending on your body weight), and working out every day for at least 45 minutes.

Is it possible? ABSOLUTELY! Whether you do it or not, check out the plan and try it in your life. I'm sure you will feel the benefits.

Day 1

Breakfast

- 1 bowl of oatmeal, not the instant variety, sprinkled with a half a teaspoon of cinnamon.
- A half a cup of blueberries
- Two tablespoons of sunflower seeds
- One small tub of natural, full fat yoghurt
- 1 cup of green tea without milk or sugar

Snack

- 200g cottage cheese
- 1 slice whole-grain bread

Lunch

- 1 whole-meal wrap
- 1 cooked chicken breast
- 1 tomato
- As much lettuce as you like
- Half an avocado

Snack

- An apple
- A handful of almonds

Dinner

- Grilled steak
- 1 potato served with a tablespoon of butter
- A salad made of baby spinach leaves, half an onion, 12 cherry tomatoes and 10 olives

Day 2

Breakfast

- A 2 egg omelet fried with one teaspoon butter; filled with grilled mushrooms
- Half an avocado

Snack

- 1 small tub natural yoghurt with ½ teaspoon cinnamon mixed in
- 1 peach

Lunch

- Portion of tuna in brine
- 1 slice whole-grain bread
- 1 teaspoon butter
- 1 green salad with a tablespoon of olive oil dressing

Snack

- 10 baby carrots
- 50g home-made hummus

Dinner

- 1 chicken breast, stir fried in 1 tablespoon olive oil with a cup of frozen stir-fry vegetables, seasoned with a dash of cayenne pepper
- 60g brown rice, cooked
- 1 cup strawberries for dessert

Day 3

Breakfast

- 2 eggs scrambled, fried in a teaspoon of butter
- 1 tomato, sliced and fried
- 230g Portobello mushrooms, brushed with balsamic vinegar and grilled
- ½ an avocado

Snack

- 2 tablespoons of Macadamia nuts
- 1 pear

Lunch

- A salad made from romaine lettuce, shredded cabbage, ½ cup watercress, ½ a mango and dressed with 1 tablespoon of olive oil mixed with 1 tablespoon of balsamic vinegar
- 1 smoked chicken breast, shredded

Snack

- 1 small tub of natural yoghurt
- 3 fresh apricots

Dinner

- 1 portion grilled salmon
- ¼ teaspoon of wasabi paste
- 1 tablespoon mayonnaise
- 2 slices wholegrain toast
- Lettuce to taste
- ¼ onion and ¼ red pepper, sliced thinly

Day 4

Breakfast

- 2 rashers back bacon, fried in a little bit of water
- 1 grilled tomato, drizzled with 1 tablespoon olive oil
- 1 small potato, boiled and then diced up and fried with half an onion in the bacon fat till crispy
- 1 slice whole-grain toast

Snack

- 2 hardboiled eggs

Lunch

- 1 large Greek salad made up of lettuce, tomato, 10 olives and 1 portion feta cheese, no dressing

Snack

- 200g cottage cheese mixed with ½ cup fresh pineapple

Dinner

- 200g Quinoa, cooked in homemade chicken stock
- Boiled mixed vegetables, served with 1 teaspoon butter
- 1 pork chop, grilled

Day 5

Breakfast

- 2 apples sliced and cored sprinkled with a crust made of ½ cup of raw oats mixed with enough butter so that it makes a crumble, sprinkled with 2 tablespoons chopped pecan nuts and ½ teaspoon cinnamon. Bake until top is crunchy.
- Serve with 1 tub natural yoghurt to which you have added 1 teaspoon honey

Snack

- Homemade guacamole
- ½ whole-grain pita bread

Lunch

- A 2 egg omelet made with 10 sliced olives and a small portion feta cheese

- 1 green salad, no dressing

Snack

- An apple
- 2 tablespoons of pistachios

Dinner

- Grilled pork tenderloin
- Vegetables sprinkled with 1 tablespoon olive oil and roasted in oven

Day 6

Breakfast

- ½ bowl cooked oatmeal mixed with ½ cup oat bran and 1 tablespoon fresh cream and sprinkled with cinnamon and 2 tablespoons walnuts
- Sliced strawberries
- 1 tub natural yoghurt

Snack

- 1 portion cheddar cheese
- 1 pear

Lunch

- 1 chicken breast, shredded
- ½ whole-meal pita bread
- ¼ cup fresh pineapple sliced
- Lettuce and tomato to taste

- Dressing made of 1 tablespoon of olive oil mixed with 1 tablespoon balsamic vinegar and a teaspoon of Dijon mustard

Snack

- ½ portion tuna in brine
- 1 slice whole-grain toast

Dinner

- 1 large lettuce leaf, stuffed with 1 tablespoon hummus and a portion of smoked salmon. Add in tomato, cucumber and sliced red pepper to taste. Serve with 4 chopped Brazil nuts.

Day 7

Breakfast

- Two slices French toast made up with two eggs (add a little milk if necessary) and fried in butter.
- Serve with ½ cup blueberries mixed with 2 tablespoons of toasted pecan nuts.

Snack

- Baby carrots and cucumber sticks
- 2 tablespoons of sunflower seeds

Lunch

- 1 wholegrain pita bread spread with a tablespoon of basil pesto and topped with sliced red and green pepper, diced tomato and 1 portion cheese.

Snack

- 1 green salad with 1 diced hardboiled egg added in
- 2 tablespoons pumpkin seeds

Dinner

- 1 steak, brushed with olive oil and black pepper and pan-fried
- 1 cup spinach, chopped and wilted with two tablespoons of fresh cream
- 1/2 cup pumpkin, roasted
- 100g mushrooms, fried in a little butter with garlic

Module 3

Breakfast Recipes

There are two main reasons while you should pay serious attention to what you eat for breakfast: First, morning is the best time to jumpstart your metabolism; Second, if you feed your body with good, balanced diet, you will be able to accomplish your weight loss goals.

Outlined below are highly effective breakfast recipes for losing weight. Each recipe is unique in its own constituents and dietary significance. You do not need to eat the same recipe every day; of course, going for a variety of foods will be a better option. Always aim to get at least 5 grams of fibers or resistance starch into your body every morning. If you can, prefer to go for home-made food and drinks. And it is quite advisable to switch from caffeinated drinks to green tea.

Blueberry Oat Pancakes with Maple Yogurt

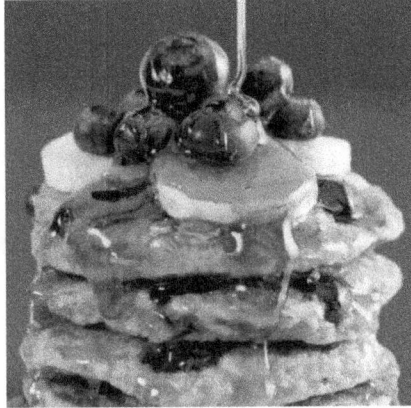

Ingredients

- Blueberries
- Low-fat yogurt
- Maple syrup
- Oats
- Low-fat cheese
- Vanilla extract
- Cooking spray
- Eggs

Calories: About 410
Resistant starch (fiber): 4.6g
Additional Comments: This breakfast contains almost 5g of resistant starch (fiber) and its ingredients are non-fat, with low risk of cholesterol.

Breakfast Barley with Banana and Sunflower Seeds

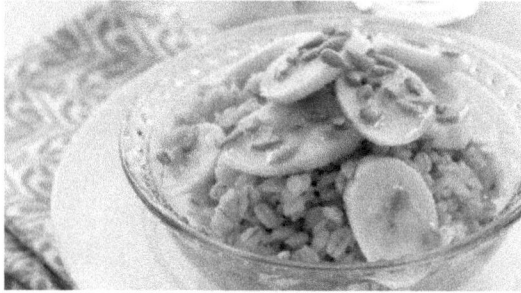

Ingredients

- Honey
- Water
- Banana
- Pearl barley
- Sunflower seeds.

Calories: About 410
Resistant starch (fiber): 7.6g
Additional Comments: The sunflower seeds are rich in fibers and protein, as well as pearl barley.

Banana and Almond Butter Toast

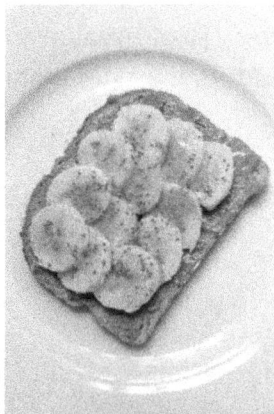

Ingredients

- Banana
- Rye bread
- Almond butter

Calories: About 280
Resistant starch (fiber): 5.6g
Additional Comments: This breakfast contains almost 5.6g of resistant starch (fiber) and its ingredients are non-fat, with very low risk of cholesterol.

Oatmeal

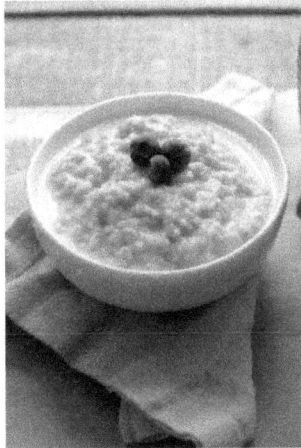

According to several studies on nutrition, having oatmeal for breakfast proffers some amazing benefits. Apart from the fact that it contains a high percentage of fiber, oatmeal reduces the level of blood sugar in human body and fights every pound of fat in your body. After consuming oatmeal, you will feel heavy, an experience that will keep you away from over-eating. Since oatmeal fights the production of insulin in human body, it keeps the amount of insulin-inspired fat storage in your body to the barest minimum.

Poached Eggs on Watercress

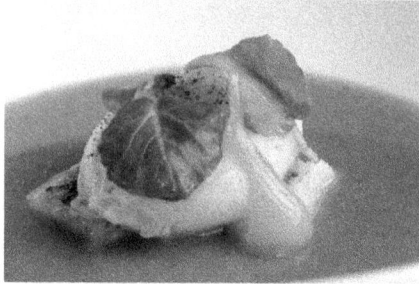

Eggs are a delicious, protein-packed super food. They are low in calories, very versatile and highly nutritious. Cooked in a low-fat way, eggs will give you enough great energy to get you through a busy morning, along with some serious nutrients. Eggs contain vitamins A, B2, B5, B12, B6, D, E and K, plus folate, selenium, calcium and zinc and served with some fresh healthy watercress and tomatoes they taste great too!

Ingredients

- 2 small free-range eggs
- A handful of watercress
- A ripe tomato
- 1 drop of vinegar
- 1 pinch of salt (for the water only)

Method

1. First, get the eggs poaching. Put on a medium-sized saucepan of water to boil and add a pinch of salt to it. Make sure your eggs are really fresh and crack each one into its own ramekin or cup. Add a small drop of vinegar to both eggs.

2. When the water is boiling, take a hand-held balloon whisk and stir the water to create a gentle whirlpool in the water, which will help the egg white wrap around the yolk.

3. Slowly tip one egg into the water, white first. As the white starts to turn opaque, crack in the other egg. Turn the heat right down to the minimum setting. Leave to cook for three minutes.

4. Meanwhile, rinse the watercress and shake it dry. Arrange a generous bed of it on a dinner plate. Slice up the tomato into narrow wedges and arrange on top of the cress. After three minutes, remove the eggs with a slotted spoon, snipping off any straggly edges using the edge of the spoon.

5. Rest each egg to drain on kitchen paper for a few seconds – this is an important step as a waterlogged dish is unpleasant. Place the egg onto the watercress and tomato bed, season and enjoy this delicious hot-cold breakfast salad.

Rainbow Zinger

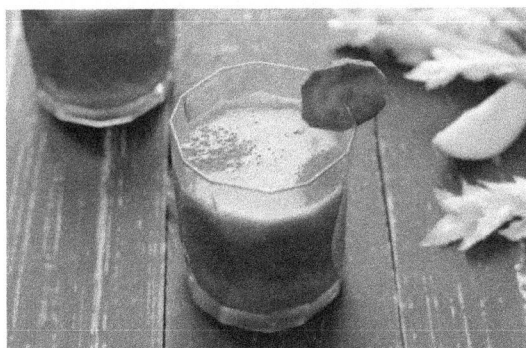

This blend of citrus fruits and root vegetables creates a lovely sweet and sour flavored juice. The Rainbow Zinger delivers lots of vitamin C, helps to cleanse your system and gives you an energy boost.

Ingredients

- 1 large lemon
- 1 lime
- 2 beetroots
- 2 carrots
- 2 apples
- A thumb-sized piece of ginger

Method

1. For this recipe you will need a juicer, or if you don't have one, blend and sieve out the juice by pressing the pulp. Peel the lemons and limes and chop the other ingredients. Place them all into the juicer and serve the drink over ice.

Smoked Salmon and Eggs Supreme

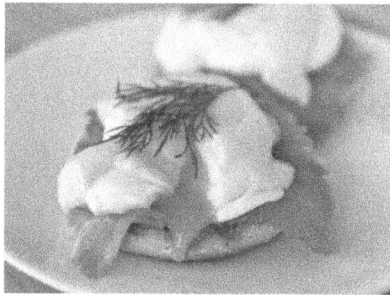

This delicious breakfast contains low-fat, high-protein smoked salmon and scrambled eggs to give you a perfectly low-fat protein hit. The nutritious eggs are enhanced by the B vitamins, vitamin D, magnesium, selenium, DHA, EPA and there are omega-3 fatty acids in the salmon.

Ingredients

- 2 large eggs

- 1 thin slice smoked salmon, diced
- Few leaves of chopped fresh spinach
- 1 splash of fat-free milk
- 1 tsp. reduced-fat cream cheese
- Low-calorie cooking spray
- 1 tsp. chopped chives
- 1 pinch freshly ground black pepper

Method

1. Mist some of the cooking spray into a medium nonstick skillet and turn it onto a medium heat. Whisk the eggs, milk and pepper a bowl until well combined. Pour the egg mixture into the skillet and cook until the mixture begins to thicken, continuously stirring it with wooden spoon. Stir in the salmon and cream cheese and cook for 30 seconds.

2. Stir in the spinach for cook 2 more minutes or until spinach wilts and the eggs are just cooked, stirring constantly. Spoon the egg and salmon mixture onto a plate and garnish with the chives, then enjoy.

Crunchy Pomegranate Yogurt

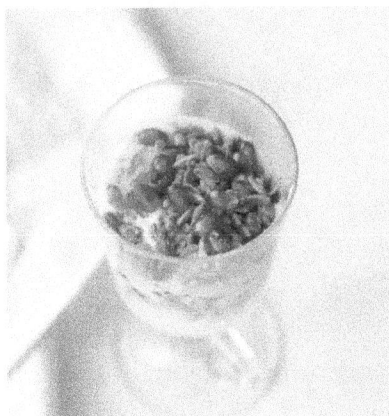

Enjoy the delicious taste of pomegranate, mixed into this tasty crunchy, creamy treat. Pomegranates are a super-powerful anti-oxidant, even more so than green tea! The pretty ruby-like seeds are sweet and juicy, plus they offer a great boost of vitamins C, E and K. Serve cold and enjoy a virtuous but memorably moreish breakfast.

Ingredients

- 1 pot of fat-free yoghurt, well chilled
- 1 pomegranate
- 1 tsp. organic oat bran
- 1 tsp. mixed seeds

Method

1. First, collect all the pomegranate seeds. One of the easiest ways to do this is to cut it in half and tap hard with a spoon so the red seeds fall into a bowl. Be careful to avoid the bitter pith. Mix the fresh pomegranate seeds with the fat-free yogurt and sprinkle over the oat bran and mixed seeds.

Superberry Smoothie

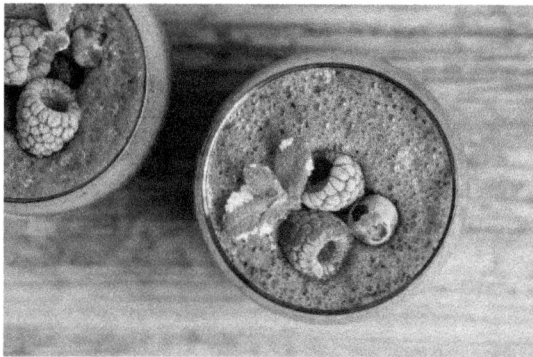

Blueberries are famously an anti-oxidant super food and cranberries are great for your health, particularly your 'waterworks'. Add some vitamin-packed raspberries and enjoy a tasty, sweet, weight-loss treat that will boost your immunity and may lower blood your pressure too.

Ingredients

- 200ml cranberry juice
- 100g blueberries
- 100g raspberries
- 100ml 1% milk
- 200ml fat-free natural yogurt
- Mint sprigs, to serve

Method

1. Place all the ingredients apart from the mint into a blender and pulse until smooth. Pour the smoothie into a tall glass and serve topped with the fresh mint.

Veggie Breakfast Bake

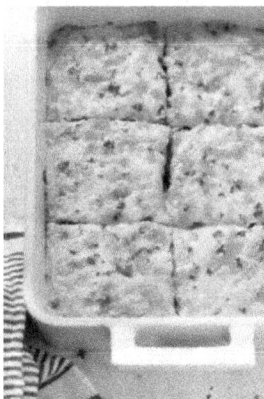

This is a delectable, vegetarian-friendly take on a cooked breakfast, with no fatty, processed bacon to pile on the calories. It features lycopene-rich tomatoes, iron-rich spinach and a lovely, tasty B-vitamin packed mushroom too. Although this is a satisfying dish, the main ingredients contain very few calories, which will help with healthy weight loss.

Ingredients

- 1 large egg
- 1 large field mushroom
- 2 tomatoes, halved
- A large handful of spinach
- 1/2 garlic clove, thinly sliced
- 1 tsp. olive oil

Method

1. Heat oven to 200C/180C fan/gas 6. Put the mushroom, tomatoes and slices of garlic into an ovenproof dish. Drizzle over the oil and grind over pepper, then bake for 10 minutes.

2. Meanwhile, put the spinach into a colander, then pour over a kettle of boiling water to wilt it. Squeeze out any excess water, then add the spinach to the dish. Make a little gap between the vegetables and crack an egg into each dish. Return to the oven and cook for a further 8-10 minutes or until the egg is cooked to your liking.

Superfood Muesli

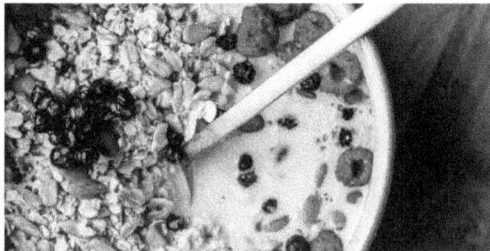

Muesli can be a great breakfast, but when you are trying to lose weight it is best to stick to a low-fat, homemade version. Store-bought muesli can be packed with hidden sugar, often in the form of too much dried fruit. Make this version and you know exactly what you are getting – heart-healthy oats, nutrient-rich nuts, goji berries which boast all 18 amino acids and some of the most potent antioxidant power known to man, plus super-healthy seeds.

Ingredients

- 2 tbsp. whole oats
- 3 almonds, roughly crushed
- 3 hazelnuts, roughly crushed
- 1 tsp. goji berries
- 1 tsp. sunflower seeds
- 1 tsp. golden flax seeds
- 200ml organic coconut milk or fat-free organic milk

Method

1. Take a large breakfast bowl and place in all the dry ingredients. Pour over the coconut or fat-free milk and stir. Leave the muesli to soak and swell for 20 minutes, then enjoy.

Spring Eggs

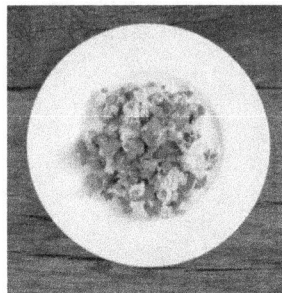

Scrambled eggs are a light but filling treat. Protein is excellent for building lean muscle and encouraging weight loss, plus it is satisfying to eat. Pep up with vitamins from the lycopene-rich tomatoes and add flavor with fresh herbs.

Ingredients

- 2 large organic eggs
- 1 medium ripe tomato
- 1 splash of fat-free milk
- 1 tsp. olive oil
- Sprig of fresh, flat-leaf parsley
- Sprig of fresh basil

Method

1. Break the eggs into a bowl. Add a splash of milk and season, then beat the mixture with a fork. Heat the oil in a skillet on a low heat and while it is warming chop the tomato into a fine dice. Pour the egg mixture into the skillet and keep stirring. Just as the eggs are starting to set, add in the chopped tomatoes and stir lightly. Remove from the heat, spoon onto a plate and tear over the parsley and basil, then enjoy.

Green Delight Smoothie

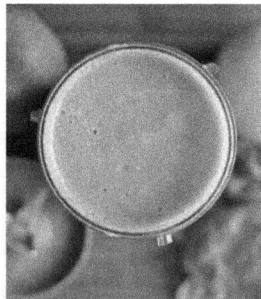

This gorgeous green smoothie features super-leaf kale, which is bursting with calcium, antioxidants and purifying compounds to help you lose both the toxins and the pounds. If you are a green smoothie-lover, you will really enjoy this healthy shot of liquid greens, softened by the sweetness of the fruit. Perfect for when you are after a totally healthy breakfast, perhaps when you are rushing off to work, or preparing for a burst of exercise soon afterwards.

Ingredients

- ¾ cup chopped kale, ribs and thick stems removed
- 1 stalk celery, chopped
- ½ small banana
- ½ cup unsweetened apple juice
- 1 tablespoon fresh lemon juice
- ½ cup ice

Method

1. Place the kale, celery, banana, apple juice, ice, and lemon juice in a blender. Blend until smooth and frothy then drink it nice and cold.

Green Glade Omelet

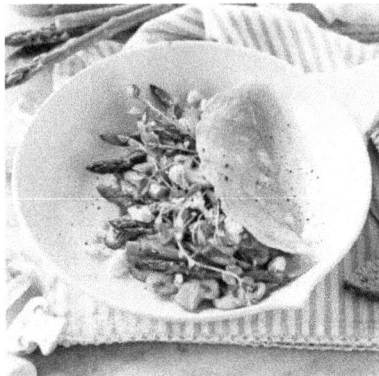

A wonderfully satisfying breakfast or brunch, especially in the fall or winter. Mushrooms, asparagus and eggs are all wholesome and low-calorie ingredients that offer a wide-variety of exceptional nutrients. All of these ingredients, when combined and given a touch of pizzazz, create a hugely enjoyable breakfast.

Ingredients

- 1/4 cup chopped, fresh asparagus
- 1/4 cup sliced mushrooms
- 1 large egg
- 3 large egg whites
- 1 tbsp. fat-free milk
- 1 small pinch of salt
- A dash of black pepper
- 1/4 cup reduced-fat mozzarella cheese (1/2 ounce)

Method

1. Put a small, nonstick skillet onto a medium-high to heat and mist with low-calorie cooking spray until it is evenly coated. Fry the asparagus and mushrooms for four minutes, or until tender. Remove them and set aside on a warm plate. Whisk the egg, egg whites, milk, salt and pepper together in a small bowl. Pour the egg mixture into the pan, coating the entire bottom of the pan and allow to cook for 2 minutes.

2. Sprinkle the cheese, mushrooms, and asparagus on one half of the omelet. Use a spatula to fold one end of the omelet over the other, so that all the vegetables are enveloped inside. Continue cooking for 2 more minutes, until egg is fully cooked through. Slide the omelet onto a plate and eat immediately.

Lunch Recipes

It is advisable you choose lunches that won't only provide you some extra energy to handle the tediousness of work in your workplace, but you should also consider the implications of your choice on your overall health. Some people always complain about lack of time for a good lunch and eventually end up in fast food restaurants. Consuming burgers and other fatty foods will only compound your weight concerns. So, if you are anxious about maintaining a healthy body or lose the current weight that has driven you into self-loathing individual, please consider settling for any the following weight-loss lunch recipes. Ok, let's get down to it.

Tuna-Avocado Sandwich

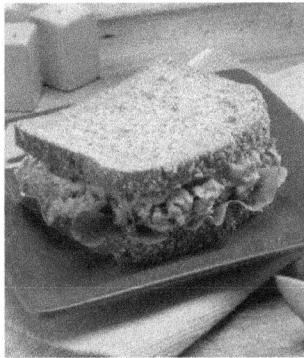

Ingredients

- 1/3 Avocado, to be mashed
- 1/2 tablespoon of lemon juice
- 4 ounces of white albacore tuna, to be drained
- 1 slice of whole-grain bread
- 1 piece of butter lettuce
- 1 thick slice of tomato
- 1 slice of red onion

Calories: 350

Additional Comments: Make a delicious tuna-Avocado sandwich with the ingredients described above. Avocados are common sources of Vitamin B and unsaturated fat, which helps lower the cholesterol in the body and prevent heart diseases. Whole grains are rich in fibers.

Tofu Salad

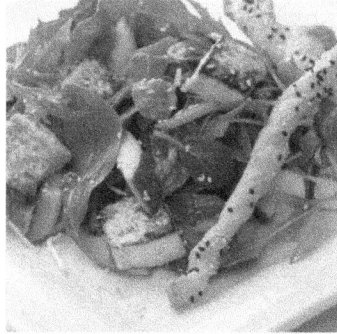

Ingredients

- 1 tablespoon of soy sauce
- 1 tablespoon of Almond butter
- 1/8 teaspoon of minced garlic
- 4 ounce of tofu, which is extra firm but thinly sliced
- 2 Scandinavian crisp bread crackers
- 1 cup of snow peas that have been slivered
- 1/2 teaspoon of sesame seeds

Calories: 330

Method

1. Whisk the soy sauce, almond butter and garlic. Throw in tofu and snow peas. Then cover with sesame seeds and serve with crackers. Almond butter is very rich in unsaturated fat.

Sesame seeds and tofu will provide the much-need fiber. The Scandinavian crisp bread crackers are rich in fiber, too.

2. If you cannot lay your hand on the suggested crackers, you can use the commonest ones in your locality. The emphasis here is that you should avoid deep-fried crackers that contain high-calories fat.

Spicy Chicken Salad

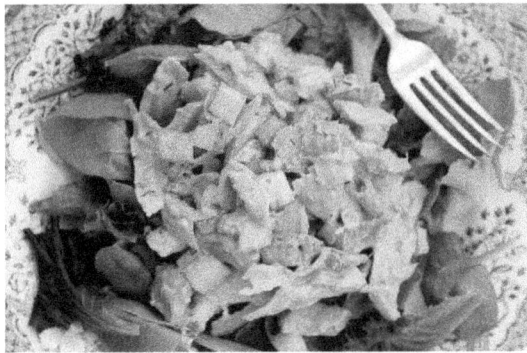

Ingredients

- 1 tablespoon of fresh lemon juice
- 1/2 jalapeno, which has been diced
- 1/2 medium celery stalk chopped into pieces
- 1 cup of roasted, cubed and skinless chicken breast
- 4 teaspoons of Dijon mustard
- 1 cup of baby spinach
- Dash of black pepper

Calories: 226

Additional Comments: Put all the ingredients together and eat them on the spinach. The capsaicin in spicy pepper will help you melt the fat in your body. Do not hesitate to replace any of the foreign or unavailable ingredients with other similar ingredients in your locality.

Mozzarella & Tomato Salad

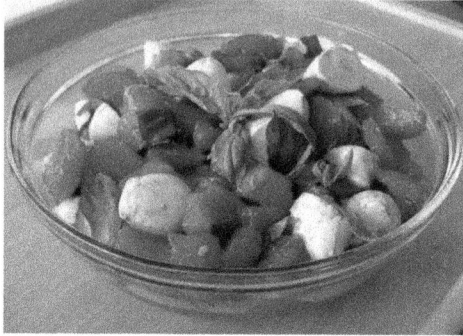

Ingredients

- 1/4 teaspoon of black pepper
- 2 tablespoons of balsamic vinegar
- 1 medium tomato that is cubed
- 2 teaspoons of sunflower seeds
- 1 clove garlic that has been pressed
- 1 ounce of fresh part-skim mozzarella cheese, cubed
- 1 1/2 teaspoon of olive oil
- 1 cup of fresh spinach leaves

Calories: 243

Additional Comments: Combine all the ingredients listed above and eat together. For the fact that it is a low-calorie lunch, it is highly recommendable for anyone willing to shed some weight within a short period of time.

Open-Faced Lox Sandwich

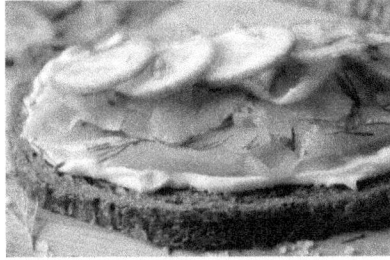

Ingredients

- 1 1/2 tablespoon of minced onions
- 2 tablespoons of capers
- 1 slice of pumpernickel bread
- 4 ounces of smoked salmon
- 2 tablespoons of part-trim ricotta

Calories: 250

Additional Comments: Grab the bread and layer other ingredients above in the order you want. This meal is delicious and it is rich with nutrients that are necessary for your body growth.

Tuna Niçoise Wrap

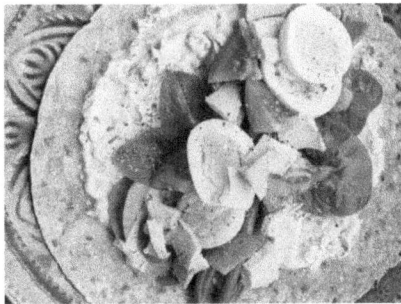

Tuna is fabulous for weight loss and heart health, being full of omega-3 fatty acids, potassium, selenium, vitamin B12 and more. The light yogurt dressing is an outstanding treat too.

Ingredients

- 1 whole-wheat or spelt pita
- 1 small can of tuna
- 1 handful fresh baby spinach leaves

For the dressing (makes enough for at least two wraps)

- ½ cup fat-free Greek yogurt
- 2 tbsp. olive oil
- 2 tbsp. lemon juice
- 1 clove garlic, pressed
- 1 pinch each salt and pepper
- ¼ cup grated parmesan cheese

Method

1. Beat all the Caesar dressing ingredients together with a fork in a bowl. Cut the pita bread to make a pocket and stuff it with the tuna and baby spinach. Spoon over half the yogurt Caesar dressing and enjoy (the remaining dressing will keep in the fridge for a few days).

Greek Salad Light

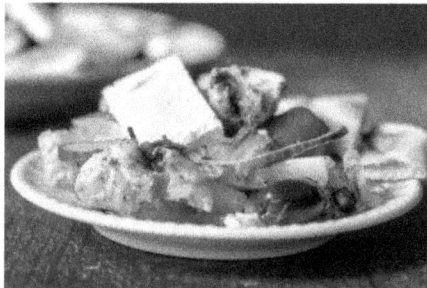

This tasty little lunch comprises all the elements of a classic Greek salad – olives, tomatoes and cucumber, but instead of feta we are using super-light cottage cheese. Olives can be fantastic for dieters. They contain healthy fats, vitamin E and minerals, but also because their strong, distinctive flavor helps to take the edge of hunger, leaving you feeling satisfied.

Ingredients

- A quarter of an iceberg lettuce, torn into pieces
- 8-10 pitted olives, chopped in half
- 2 medium tomatoes, diced
- ¼ cucumber, diced
- 3 tbsp. low-fat cottage cheese
- A few leaves of fresh basil

Method

1. Scatter the lettuce onto a plate and spoon the cottage cheese, cucumber and tomato over them, sprinkled with the olives and torn basil, then enjoy.

Shrimp and Fennel Salad with Citrus Dressing

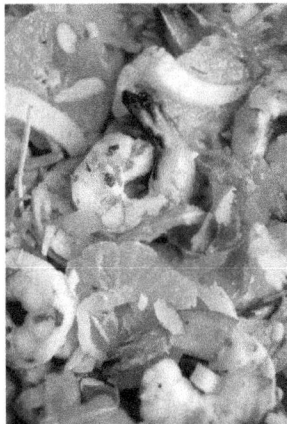

Freshly cooked shrimp and be an exceptional, low-calorie treat. Shrimp are superb seafood, very nutritious, with selenium astaxathin, an antioxidant and anti-inflammatory nutrient. Selenium helps to ensure a strong thyroid function, essential for anyone who wishes to control their weight.

Ingredients

- 3 oz. raw shrimp
- A large handful of mixed lettuce leaves
- ¼ cup chopped fennel
- 1/3 avocado, sliced
- 1 tbsp. lemon juice
- 1 tsp. olive oil
- Juice of half an orange, plus segments of the other half
- Juice of half a pink grapefruit, plus segments of the other half
- 1 garlic clove
- 2 tsp. sunflower seeds
- 2 tsp. Parmesan shavings
- Low-calorie cooking spray

Method

1. Sauté the shrimp with the crushed garlic and lemon juice in a skillet coated with the low-calorie cooking spray. Combine the lettuce and the chopped fennel.

2. Whisk together the olive oil and citrus juice, then toss the dressing together with the mixed greens, avocado, shrimp and citrus segments. Top with the Parmesan shavings and sunflower seeds.

Chicken and Avocado Salad

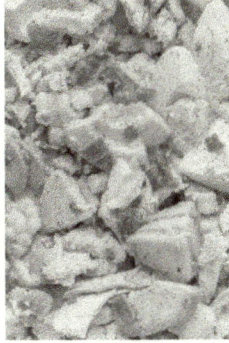

Chicken is a great and tasty source of lean protein, while avocado is an excellent source of healthy fats that are good for the skin and organs. Both can help to promote weight loss when eaten as part of a balanced diet and this particular recipe is so simple and delicious that it is bound to become a family favorite.

Ingredients

- 1 skinless chicken breast
- 2 tsp. olive oil (1 for the salad)
- 1 heaped tsp. smoked paprika

For the salad

- ½ small ripe avocado, diced
- 1 tsp. red wine vinegar
- 1 tbsp. flat-leaf parsley, roughly chopped
- 1 medium tomato, chopped
- ½ small red onion, thinly sliced

Method

1. Heat grill to medium. Rub the chicken all over with 1 tsp. of the olive oil and the paprika. Cook for 4-5 minutes each side until lightly charred and cooked through.

2. Mix the salad ingredients together, season and add the rest of the oil. Thickly slice the chicken and serve with salad.

Chicken and Soba Noodle Soup

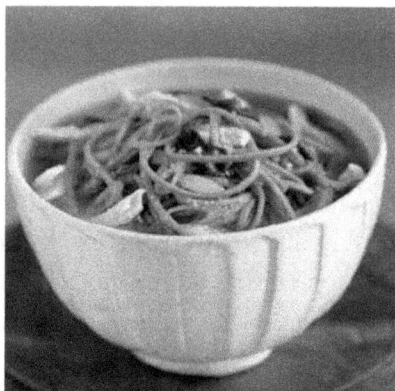

Sometimes, in the middle of the day you just need a light but hearty, warming soup. Soba noodles are a great lower carb option for this recipe, the chicken gives the lean protein hit and the oriental vegetables will also help to fill you up for the rest of the day, all for very few calories.

Ingredients

- 500ml vegetable stock
- 85g cooked chicken, shredded
- A handful of mixed Chinese vegetables: beansprouts, sweet corn, water chestnuts, sliced carrot and mange tout
- 80g dried soba noodles
- 2 spring onions, sliced, to serve
- A thumb-sized piece fresh root ginger, grate
- 1 garlic clove, grated
- 2 tsp. soy sauce and 2 tsp. sugar
- Juice of 1 lime

Method

1. Cook the soba noodles according to the packet instructions. Put stock, ginger, garlic, soy sauce and sugar in a saucepan, then heat. Simmer for 5 minutes. Take off the heat, pour into a microwave-safe bowl, then cool. Throw in the chicken and vegetables, cover, then chill for a few hours or up to a day.

2. When ready to eat, remove from fridge, then add the cooked noodles. Microwave on high for 2 minutes, stir, then cook for 1 minute more or until piping hot. Divide between two bowls, sprinkle with the sliced spring onions and add the lime juice.

Tomato Quinoa Tabbouleh

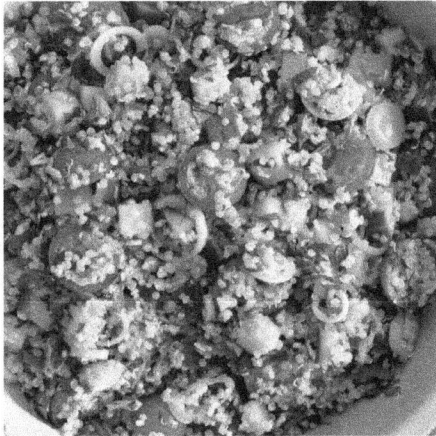

Quinoa is a high-protein grain that makes tasty salads, pilafs, side dishes and much more. It goes beautifully with low-calorie tomatoes, parsley and cucumber for the perfect, meat-free but fresh and filling weight loss lunch.

Ingredients

- 100g dried quinoa

- 75g parsley, roughly chopped
- 300g ripe tomatoes, cut into 1cm dice
- 100g cucumber, cut into small dice

For the dressing

- 1 tbsp. olive oil
- 2 tbsp. balsamic vinegar
- Juice and zest of ½ lemon
- Drop of vanilla extract
- 1 tsp. rice syrup or agave
- Pinch of salt
- ½ garlic clove, crushed
- 50g salad leaves, to serve

Method

1. Cook the quinoa following pack instructions, then set aside to cool.

2. Make the dressing by adding the olive oil, vinegar, lemon juice, vanilla extract, rice syrup, pinch of salt and garlic into a jug and whisk until smooth.

3. Mix the dressing into the quinoa and then mix together with all the other ingredients. Serve on a bed of salad leaves.

Ham and Beets Bowl

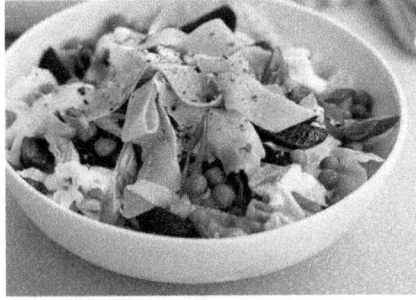

Ham can be something we crave when trying to lose weight. But unlike other forms of pork, lean ham can be the perfect choice as it is possible to buy a really low-fat product. The sweetness of the meat, peas and beets makes this a really lovely, enjoyable dish, packed with lean protein and fiber.

Ingredients

- 100g wafer-thin sliced ham
- Half an iceberg lettuce, shredded
- 100g frozen peas
- 175g beets
- 2 spring onions, thinly sliced
- 2 tbsp. fat-free Greek yogurt
- 2 tsp. horseradish sauce

Method

1. Pour boiling water over the peas and leave for 2 minutes, then drain well. Chop the beetroot into cubes.

2. Tip the peas, beetroot and spring onions into a bowl and mix well. Mix the yogurt and horseradish, and add about 1 tbsp. boiling water to make a pouring sauce. Pile the lettuce into bowls, and spoon over the beetroot mix. Thinly drizzle the dressing over the salad and top with ham.

Lean Turkey Tortillas

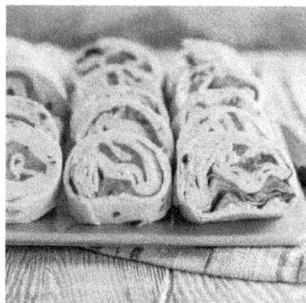

As poultry goes, turkey has to be among the leanest of protein options. One 5oz serving contains 90 calories against chickens 165 calories and typically holds just a fifth of the fat. This recipe is a super-quick and easy lunch choice. Go for the lowest calorie, lightest tortillas you can find and you're on your way!

Ingredients (Serves 4)

- 250g cooked turkey, shredded
- 4 curly lettuce leaves
- 4 whole-wheat or spelt tortillas
- 6 spring onions, shredded
- 12cm chunk cucumber, shredded
- 2 tbsp. reduced-fat mayonnaise
- 2 tbsp. pesto

Method

1. Preheat the oven to 160°C. Heat up the tortillas until they are warm but not crispy. Meanwhile, mix together the mayonnaise and pesto. Take out the warm wholegrain tortillas.

2. Divide the lettuce leaves, turkey, spring onions and cucumber between the four tortillas. Drizzle over the pesto dressing, roll up and eat.

Springtime Italian Soup

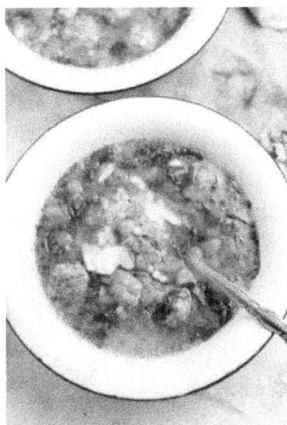

If in doubt when on a diet, go for plenty of vegetables, or soup. This brilliant recipe combines the best of both in a filling broth that boasts the addition of tasty spaghetti noodles. So delicious and full of fiber – eat up without guilt!

Ingredients

- 200g mixed green vegetables: asparagus, broad beans and spring onions
- 700ml hot vegetable stock
- 1cm-wide column of dried spaghetti
- 215g can butter beans, rinsed and drained
- 3 tbsp. green pesto

Method

1. Break up the spaghetti into inch-long pieces. In one pan, bring water to the boil and then add the spaghetti pieces.

Place the green vegetables in another saucepan, and pour over the stock. Bring to the boil, then reduce the heat and simmer until the vegetables are cooked through, about 3 minutes.

2. Stir in the cooked pasta, beans and 1 tbsp. of pesto. Warm through, then ladle into bowls and top each with another drizzle of pesto.

Thai King Prawns

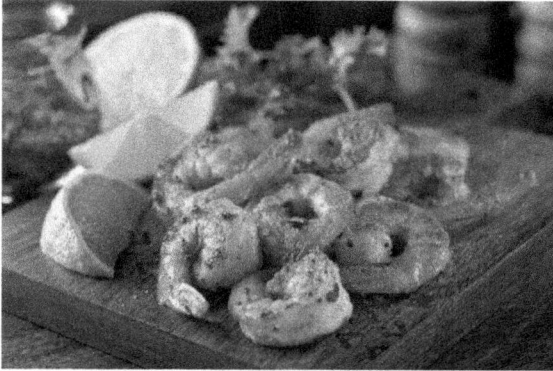

Prawns are a year-round taste sensation and this recipe, which delivers plenty of sweet, hot and sour Thai flavor, really is one of the best out there. All you are eating here is super-lean protein with nutrients, chili to speed up your metabolism and plenty of fiber, all given an oriental punch thanks to the fabulous flavors. What more could you wish for in a delicious, low-calorie, fat-busting lunch?

Ingredients (Serves 4)

- 20 raw king prawns
- 1 small shallot, finely chopped
- 4 garlic cloves, finely chopped
- 1 fresh red chili, halved, seeded and finely chopped
- 2½ cm piece of fresh root ginger, peeled and finely chopped

- 1 stem of lemongrass, tough outer leaves removed, finely chopped
- A good handful of fresh mint leaves, finely chopped
- A good handful of fresh coriander leaves, finely chopped
- 100ml olive oil
- Grated zest and juice of 1 lime
- Two large handfuls of watercress to serve

Method

1. Tip all the chopped ingredients into a bowl. Add the olive oil along with the lime zest and juice and mix well. Set aside for 30 minutes to allow the flavors to mingle.

2. To make fragrant Thai prawns, remove heads and peel shells from 20 raw king prawns but leave tail sections on. Toss the prawns in the marinade and cook in a piping hot skillet, or if you are eating al fresco, on a really hot barbecue for 45 seconds on each side until they turn from grey-blue to pink.

3. Serve the hot prawns on a bed of watercress and tuck in freely to this low-calorie, low-carb, low-fat dish!

Dinner Recipes

Be selective when choosing what to eat for dinner because your body undergoes minimal metabolic activities during the night. So, you should go for food that is easily digestible. Not only that, foods that are rich in fiber and contain little or no cholesterol tend to help your body fight fatness which, according to many researches, builds up mainly while you are sleeping.

In the light of this, your dinners should be low-calorie foods. Drink as much liquid (water, tea et cetera) as you can because you may lose some water through sweating and mid-night urination. As you may have discovered in this book, keeping the water balance in your body is a task you must pay serious attention to. Because metabolic activities in human body requires a great deal of liquidity.

Baked Chicken with Mushrooms and Sweet Potato

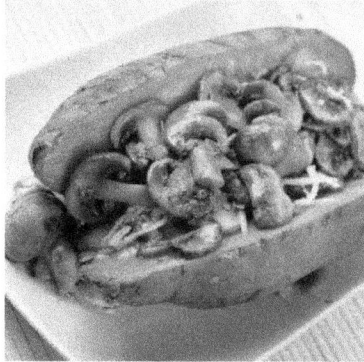

Ingredients

- 1/2 skinless chicken breast
- 1 tablespoon of olive oil
- 1 medium sweet potato
- 1 cup of sliced baby Portobello mushrooms
- 1 tablespoon of chives

Calories: 382

Method

1. Use a microwave oven set at 370°F to bake chicken with mushrooms, chives and oil as the tops for 15 minutes. Microwave potato from 5 to 7 minutes. If you cannot lay your hands on Portobello mushrooms, use the commonest and nutritious mushrooms in your locality.

Additional Comments: Potatoes normally have high fiber content, and olive oil will introduce low-cholesterol, unsaturated fat into your body. Unsaturated fat is known for preventing heart problems in human body.

Light Lasagna

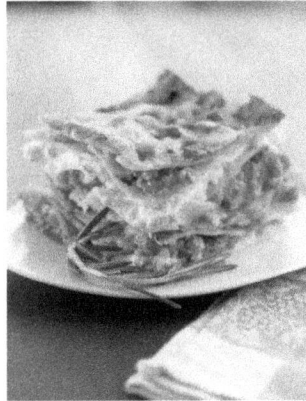

Ingredients

- 1/4 cup of part-skim ricotta
- 2 cups of spinach
- 1/3 cup of prepared tomato sauce
- 1/2 cup of cooked whole-wheat spaghetti
- 1/2 teaspoon of crushed red chili flakes
- 1 Coleman Natural Mild Italian Chicken Sausage link

Calories: 350

Method

1. Put pasta, ricotta, tomato sauce and chili flakes together and then scatter crumbled sausage on them. The next step involving wilting the food after adding spinach to it.

Additional Comments: Whole-wheat pasta is recognized as the reservoir of fibers, which is an active weight-reducing substance.

Jambalaya Blend with Veggie

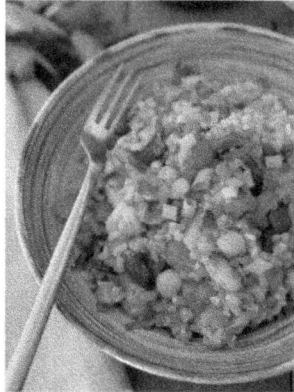

Ingredients

- 1/4 cup of chopped red onions
- 1 teaspoon of olive oil
- 1 veggie burger
- Salt
- 3/4 cup of diced zucchini
- 2 tablespoons of salsa
- 1/2 cup of brown rice
- 3/4 cup of diced squash
- 1/2 cup of chopped red, green, or yellow bell pepper
- 2 tablespoons of corn

Calories: 360

Method

1. You need to cook burger in a pan spritzed with cooking spray. Put rice, salsa, corn, salt, oil and veggies into chopped burger

and roast everything from 15 to 20 minutes. You can serve this as a side dish.

Additional Comments: Peppers are considered as a viable fat-burning substance because of capsaicin, a compound that gives it burning sensation.

Asian Snapper

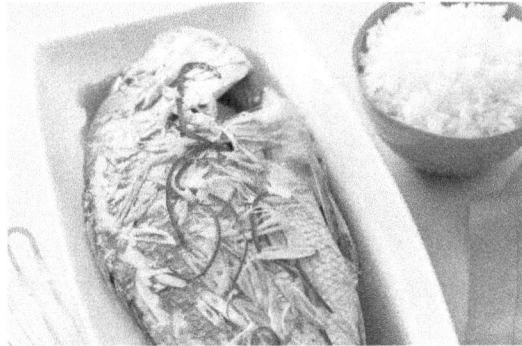

Ingredients

- 2 teaspoons of sesame seeds
- 1/2 cup of cooked millet
- 1/2 cup of cooked sugar snap peas
- 1/2 cup of raw pistachios
- 1/2 cup of bok choy
- 6 ounces of cooked snapper
- 4 teaspoons of low-sodium soy sauce

Calories: 510

Method

1. The first step is mixing millet with pistachios together. Put bok choy on top of millet and snapper. Pour soy sauce on the

snapper and then scatter sesame seeds on it. You can serve sugar snap peas as a side menu.

Additional Comments: The low-sodium soy sauce contains a vital mineral and bok choy and millet are good sources of fiber.

Cheesy Veggie Pasta

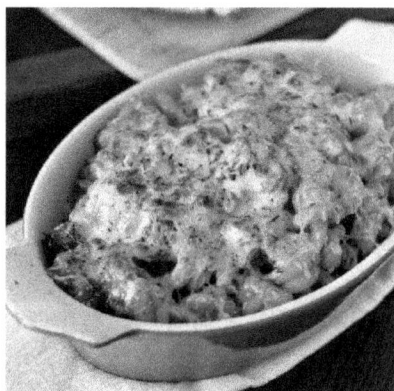

Ingredients

- 1 cup of zucchini wedges
- 1/2 cup of whole-wheat macaroni
- 2 teaspoons of olive oil
- 3/4 of chopped spinach
- 1 cup of crushed whole, peeled canned tomatoes
- 1/2 cup of low-fat ricotta cheese

Calories: 439

Method

1. First of all, cook the vegetables using medium-high heat and then mixed with cooked macaroni and cheese.

Additional Comments: Vegetables are rich in vitamins and other minerals, substances that are needed in day-to-day metabolic processes.

Black Bream with Herby Tomato Sauce

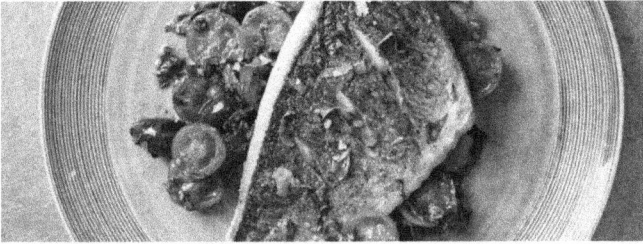

The fresh fish in this delicious dish is an outstanding low-calorie treat. Black bream makes a high protein, high-flavor basis for this easy-to-cook dish. It tastes great when cooked with a little canola oil, which has the lowest level of saturated fat of all cooking oils.

Ingredients (Serves 4)

- 4 x 6oz bream fillets, skin on
- 2 cups chopped seeded plum tomato
- 1 ½ tbsp. capers
- 1 tbsp. Dijon mustard
- 3 garlic cloves, minced
- 2 large handfuls of baby leaf spinach
- 1 ½ tbsp. chopped fresh flat-leaf parsley
- 1 ½ tbsp. minced fresh chives
- 1 tbsp. minced fresh tarragon
- 1 ½ tbsp. olive oil
- 1 tbsp. canola oil
- A large pinch of freshly ground black pepper, divided
- A pinch of salt

Method

1. Heat the olive oil in a medium skillet over medium-high heat. Add the tomato to pan and cook for 5 minutes, stirring frequently. Stir in the capers, Dijon mustard and minced garlic, allow to simmer for 3 minutes or until slightly thickened, stirring occasionally. Remove from the heat and stir in the parsley, chives, tarragon, salt and black pepper. Cover to keep warm.

2. Bring a large pan with a shallow amount of water in it to the boil. Heat the canola oil in a large nonstick skillet over medium-high heat. Season the snapper lightly with salt and black pepper and add it to the pan, skin side down.

3. In the meantime, wilt the spinach in the shallow boiling water – this will take seconds. Drain and keep warm. Cook for 3 minutes or until skin is browned, the turn the fish over; cook for a further 3 minutes or until it is as done as you like. Serve the fish on top of a bed of spinach with the sauce poured over the top of both.

Mexican Chicken and Quinoa

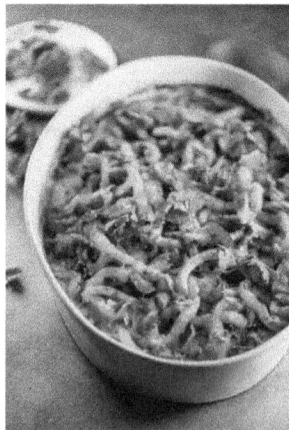

Make yourself a healthy, earthy chicken dinner. Pinto beans are a very good source of cholesterol-lowering fiber, as well as protein, folate, vitamin B1, and vitamin B6. They also contain minerals copper, phosphorus, iron, magnesium, manganese, and potassium so are truly nutrient-packed.

Ingredients (Serves 4)

- 1 tbsp. olive oil
- 1 onion, sliced
- 2 red peppers, deseeded and chopped into chunks
- 3 tbsp. chipotle paste
- 2 x 400g cans chopped tomatoes
- 4 skinless chicken breasts
- 140g quinoa
- 2 chicken stock cubes
- 1 x 400g can pinto beans, drained
- Small bunch coriander, most chopped, a few leaves left whole
- Juice 1 lime
- Fat-free natural yogurt, to serve

Method

1. Heat the oil in a deep-frying pan and fry the onions and peppers for a few minutes until softened. Stir in the chipotle paste for a minute, followed by the tomatoes.

2. Add up to a tomato can-full of water to cover the chicken and bring to a gentle simmer. Add the chicken breasts and gently simmer, turning the chicken occasionally, for 20 minutes until the chicken is cooked through.

3. Bring a large saucepan of water to the boil with the stock cubes. Add the quinoa and cook for 15 minutes until tender, adding the beans for the final minute.

4. Drain well and stir in the coriander and lime juice, then check for seasoning before covering to keep warm. Lift the chicken out onto a board and shred each breast using two forks. Stir back into the tomato sauce and season.

5. Serve with the quinoa, scattering the stew with some coriander leaves just before serving. Eat with a dollop of yogurt on the side.

Sesame Tofu Noodles

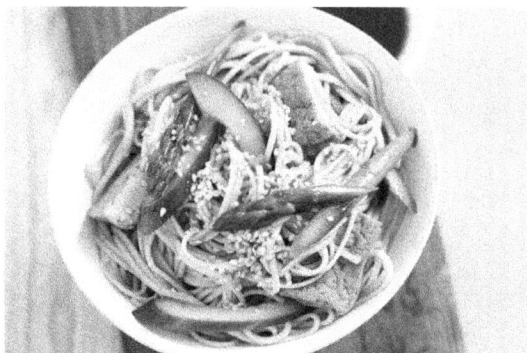

Tofu is not just for vegetarians, even though this high-protein, low-fat bean curd is a great alternative to meat. It takes on the flavors of its sauce and when cooked well it has a lovely, pleasant texture. This recipe makes a great healthy supper, full of protein and fiber as well as superb taste.

Ingredients (Serves 4)

- 250g pack firm tofu, drained
- 2 tbsp. reduced-salt soy sauce, plus extra to serve

- 300g green veg, mange tout and halved bok choy
- 300g pack straight-to-wok egg noodles
- 1 tbsp. sesame seed
- 1 tbsp. sesame oil
- 1 garlic clove, sliced
- Small knob of ginger, peeled and shredded

Method

1. Cut the tofu into bite-sized pieces and mix with 1 tbsp. of soy sauce and 1 tsp. of sesame oil. Heat the remaining oil in a wok, then stir-fry the vegetables, garlic and ginger for 2 minutes until the vegetables are starting to wilt. Drizzle with 2 tbsp. water, then stir-fry for another minute.

2. Add the noodles, sesame seeds and soy sauce from the marinated tofu, then stir-fry for 2 minutes. Now add the tofu, splash over the remaining soy sauce, and then cover with a lid. Leave for 1 minute so that the tofu heats through, then gently mix into the rest of the stir-fry. Lift the noodles and tofu into bowls and splash over a little more soy sauce then serve.

Chinese Fish Parcels

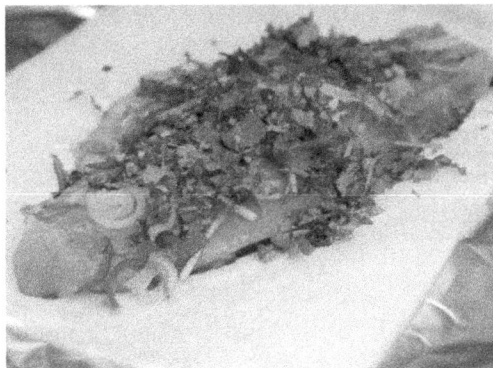

Steaming fish in a foil parcel is a great way of cooking this super-healthy protein. Treat yourself to some flavor-packed brain food with a small serving of rice and you have one super-light, healthy and warming weekday supper.

Ingredients (Serves 4)

- 4 plaice, haddock other white fish fillets
- 2 cups of rice
- 2 bok choy, thickly sliced
- 4 spring onions, shredded
- 1 red chili, thinly sliced
- 3cm ginger, cut into matchsticks
- 2 tbsp. reduced-salt soy sauce
- Juice of 1 lime
- 1 tsp. sesame oil

Method

1. Heat oven to 200C/180C fan/gas 6. Bring a pan of water to the boil. Place each fillet in the center of a large square of foil. Top each piece of fish with the bok choy, spring onions, chili and ginger, then pull up the edges of the foil. Mix together the soy sauce, lime juice and 1 tbsp. of water then spoon a little over each fillet. Place the rice in the boiling water and simmer until cooked.

2. Meanwhile, crimp the top of the foil to enclose the fish and make sure there are no gaps for the steam to escape. Place the parcels on a baking sheet and bake for 10-15 minutes until the fish is cooked through (this will depend on the thickness of your fish). Open up the parcels and drizzle over a few drops of sesame oil. Serve with the rice.

Spiced Chicken with Pomegranate Salad

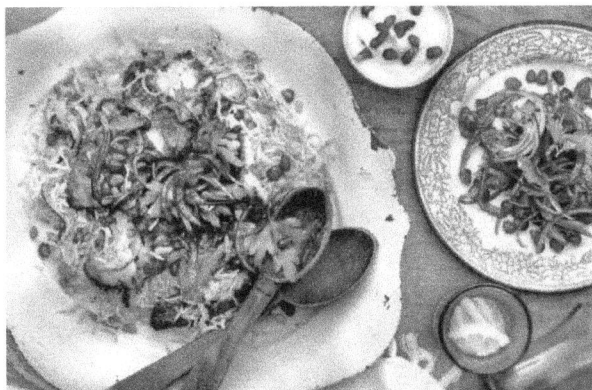

Just because you are getting your bikini body into shape, the food does not have to be boring. This delicious, Indian-inspired chicken dish packs plenty of flavors into every mouthful. It may be sweeter than some diet dishes, but because you serve it with just the salad instead of rice or potatoes you cut out the starch and keep the calories low.

Ingredients (Serves 4)

- 4 skinless chicken leg joints, cut into drumsticks and thighs
- 2½ tsp. turmeric
- 2½ tsp. sweet paprika
- ½ tsp. chili flakes
- 2½ tsp. coarsely ground black pepper
- 1 tbsp. olive oil
- 3 tbsp. white wine vinegar

For the salad

- Seeds from 1 pomegranate
- 3 oranges, segmented
- Juice ½ lime, plus extra wedges to serve

- 1 tbsp. pomegranate molasses
- Small handful mint leaves, torn

Method

1. Score the chicken with a sharp knife, about 2-3 cuts in each piece. Mix the spices with a little salt, the olive oil and vinegar in a small bowl. Using gloves (to avoid turmeric stains), rub this spice mixture over the chicken pieces and transfer to a roasting tin. Leave to marinate for at least 20 minutes, or overnight in the fridge if you're preparing ahead.

2. Heat oven to 200C/180C fan/gas 6. Cover the chicken with foil and bake for 30 minutes. Remove the foil and continue cooking in the oven for another 10 minutes until tender. Baste with tin juices and rest for 5 minutes before serving.

3. Meanwhile, make the salad. Mix the pomegranate seeds with the orange segments, mix the lime juice with the pomegranate molasses and then drizzle over. Scatter the salad with torn mint leaves and serve alongside the chicken.

Spiced Turkey Peppers

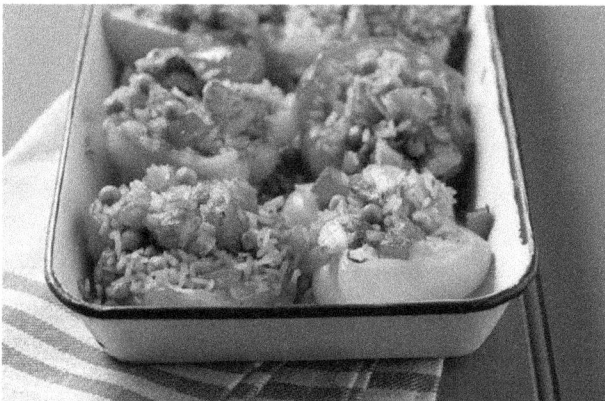

This recipe is bound to become a family favorite. The low-calorie turkey takes up all the spicy flavors of the sauce whilst remaining moist inside the pepper. It is a perfect dish when served with just a refreshing green salad on the side – the tastes and textures are so satisfying that you won't miss the rice.

Ingredients (Serves 2)

- 125g turkey mince
- 1 x 400g can plum tomatoes
- 2 red bell peppers
- 1 onion
- 1 carrot
- 1 small chili pepper
- 2 cloves garlic
- 1 tsp. cumin
- 1 tsp. olive oil
- Fresh cilantro
- 1 lime
- 2 handfuls of arugula and watercress or other salad leaves

Method

1. Pre-heat your oven to 180°C. Pour the plum tomatoes into a saucepan and break them up with a wooden spoon. Set them on a moderate heat and leave them to simmer and reduce down by about a third.

2. In the meantime, finely chop the carrot, onion, garlic and chili. Fry the chopped vegetables gently in the olive oil in a large skillet. When they are soft and sweated down, add in the turkey mince to the skillet. Keep breaking up the turkey with the wooden spoon as it cooks – you want a nice even mince, not lumps.

3. When the mince is just cooked, add the cumin and stir. Next, add the reduced plum tomatoes and coriander to the frying pan and mix well. Slice the tops of the two bell peppers about an inch down, leaving the tops intact as 'lids'. Scoop out all the seeds and white pith, then place them on a baking tray.

4. Spoon the turkey mixture into each pepper, filling them well. Pop the 'lids' back on and place the peppers in the oven for about 35 minutes. When the peppers nearly ready, dress the salad leaves with a squeeze of lime and season.

5. When you take the peppers out, they should be softened, slightly charred on top and possibly oozing juice. Serve piping hot and enjoy with your green salad.

Tuna Steak Provençal

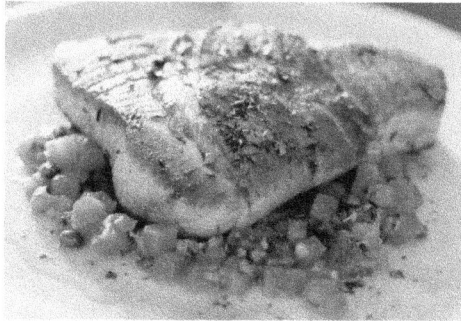

A mouthwatering recipe for when you fancy a hearty fish supper, one that goes very nicely with a few green beans. The sauce should be chunky and thick, in a rustic French style. The tomato sauce is full of nutritional treats including lycopene and the antioxidants from the tasty olives. A great weight loss dish at any time of year.

Ingredients (Serves 2)

- 2 x 150g fresh tuna steaks

- 1 x 400g can plum tomatoes
- ½ yellow bell pepper
- ½ red bell pepper
- 1 medium onion
- 10 black olives, pitted and halved
- 1 tsp. mixed dried herbs
- 2 tsp. olive oil
- A dash of Worcestershire sauce
- 2 handfuls of green beans

Method

1. Slice the onion and cut the pepper into strips. Fry them gently in half the olive oil in a medium-sized saucepan, so that they soften but do not turn brown.

2. Add the tomatoes to the onion and peppers, then add in the herbs, olives and Worcestershire sauce and leave the sauce simmering.

3. Put a small pan of water on to boil for the green beans. Heat the remaining olive oil in a large skillet. When the oil is really hot, lay in the tuna steaks.

4. Don't go away - as soon as one side seals, give it a minute and then turn it over, let that side seal and then remove it from pan to plate. Tuna is at its most delicious rare, but of course you can cook it right through if you prefer.

5. Quickly drop the green beans into the boiling water and leave for a few seconds to a minute depending on how you prefer them. Spoon the Provençal sauce over each tuna steak and serve with the green beans straight away.

Country Pork with Vegetable Medley

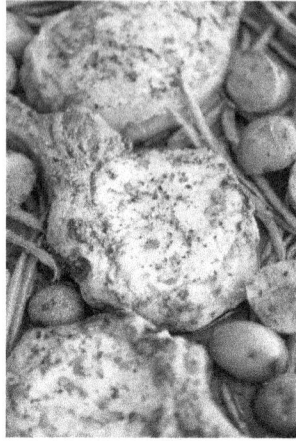

The pork in this recipe is lean and made all the more delicious by adding an apple and some low-fat crème fraîche. The freshly cooked vegetable medley makes a simple but highly nutritious and fiber-rich accompaniment.

Ingredients (Serves 2)

- 2 good-sized medallions of pork tenderloin
- 1 sweet, red apple
- 4 shallots
- 2 dessert spoons half-fat crème fraîche
- 2 tsp. olive oil
- Mixed fresh vegetables: broccoli, green beans, carrots, baby corn

Method

1. Pre-heat the oven to 200°C. Core the apple and cut it into chunky slices and place it in a small roasting tin, alongside the shallots, still in their skins. Place in the oven for twenty minutes. Meanwhile, generously season the pork medallions

with freshly ground black pepper. When the apple and shallots have been cooking for twenty minutes, take out the roasting tin, spoon the olive oil into a clear space and place the medallions on top. Place back in the oven for around another ten minutes.

2. Boil some water for the vegetables. When the pork is cooked, remove it onto a warmed plate, along with the apple and shallots. Place the vegetables in the water to cook. Place the roasting tin on a low heat on the hob and stir the crème fraîche into the pan juices.

3. Add a grinding of salt and a little hot water, ideally from vegetables that you have boiled as an accompaniment. Let the sauce bubble and thicken, then pour it over the pork medallions. Serve the vegetable medley alongside.

Asian Sirloin Salad

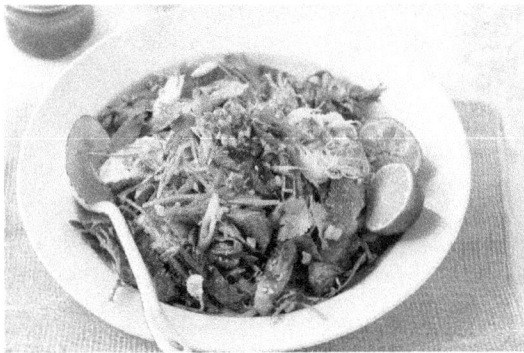

This is a great recipe for when you have company but want to stay on track in terms of weight loss. Beef can be fatty, but not this trimmed sirloin steak, which is served with lots of tempting vegetables and fresh mango so the whole protein and fiber-rich dish remains light and very tasty.

Ingredients (Serves 4)

- 3/4 pound trimmed sirloin steak (1 inch thick)
- 1 tsp. grated lime zest
- 3 tbsp. fresh lime juice
- 1 tbsp. honey
- 1 tbsp. chopped pickled ginger
- 2 tsp. low-sodium soy sauce
- 3 tbsp. canola oil
- 1 large head romaine lettuce, cut into strips (about 7 cups)
- 1 mango, cut into thin strips
- 1 red bell pepper, thinly sliced
- 1/2 cup fresh basil leaves, sliced
- 2 scallions, thinly sliced
- 1 tsp. toasted sesame seeds
- Kosher salt and black pepper

Method

1. Heat a large skillet over high heat. Season the steak with pinches of salt and black pepper. Cook 4 to 5 minutes per side for medium-rare. Let rest on a plate for at least 5 minutes before slicing.

2. Meanwhile, in a large bowl, whisk together the lime zest and juice, honey, ginger, soy sauce, oil, and a pinch of salt. Add the lettuce, mango, bell pepper, basil, and scallions and toss to combine. Finally, gently fold in the steak and sprinkle with the sesame seeds.

Malaga Fish Stew

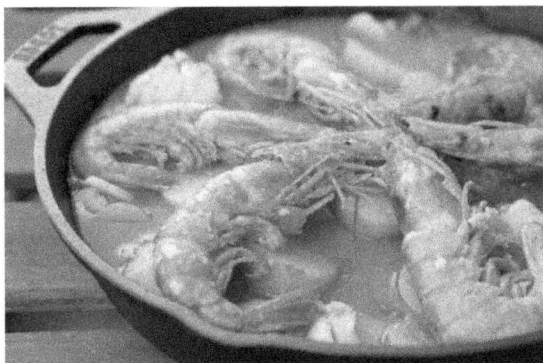

A lovely light, tasty but earthy stew, which offers lots of protein for few calories. This does not need potatoes or rice to go with it – it is very satisfying on its own, just serve it in a bowl and enjoy.

Ingredients

- 200g raw peeled king prawns
- ½ a 410g/14oz can chickpeas, rinsed and drained
- 500g thick skinless white fish fillets cut into very large chunks
- 400g can chopped tomatoes
- 3 tbsp. olive oil, plus extra to serve
- 1 medium onion, finely sliced
- 1 tsp. paprika
- A pinch of cayenne pepper
- 1 fish stock cube
- A handful of flat-leaf parsley leaves, chopped
- 2 garlic cloves, finely chopped
- Zest and juice 1 lemon

Method

1. In a small bowl, mix the parsley with ½ the garlic and lemon zest, then set aside. Heat 2 tbsp. oil in a large sauté pan. Throw in the onion and cover the pan, then sweat it for about

5 minutes until the onion has softened. Add the remaining oil, garlic and spices, and cook for 2 minutes more. Pour over the lemon juice and sizzle for a moment. Add the tomatoes, ½ a can of water and crumble in the stock.

2. Season with a little salt, and then cover the pan. Simmer everything for 5 minutes or so. Stir through the prawns and chickpeas, then ease the fish chunks into the top of the stew.

3. Reduce the heat and cover the pan, then cook for about 8 minutes, stirring very gently once or twice. When the fish is just cooked through, remove from the heat, scatter with the parsley mix and enjoy.

Snack Ideas

It is no longer a new discovery that people normally gravitate towards sweet and fatty deserts and snacks because that has been the norm or trend in the society. At every corner, sweet shops are opening in a great number serving high-calorie, high-sugar snacks and sweets to people. There is something to be worried about in this circumstance: people are getting obese and some are even suffering from type 2 diabetes.

To reverse this delicate situation, it is very important to explore a better set of snacks that are highly nutritious, low-fat, low-calories and can aid the metabolic process in human body. Below is a list of five weight-loss snacks that are actually great for your health!

Roasted Chickpeas

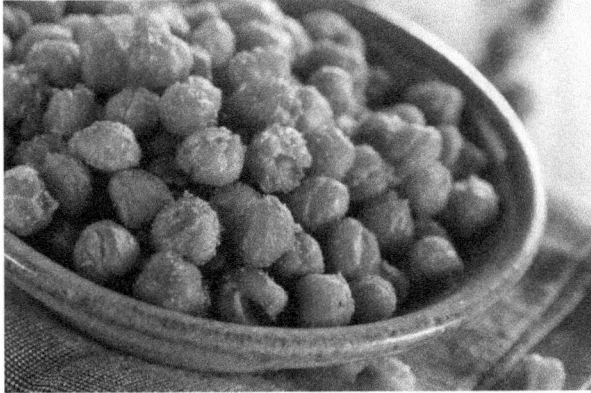

Roasted chickpeas are rich in fiber and each serve provides 5 grams of protein to your body. It is also a low-calorie snack: Imagine, 25 grams of chickpeas will only produce 95 calories!

With its composition of dietary fiber and protein, chickpeas stand out as a good snack for those who want to lose their weight in a short period of time. It is always nice if you could prepare the roasted chickpeas yourself. You can roast them by using Himalayan salt, turmeric and cayenne pepper.

A Protein Bar

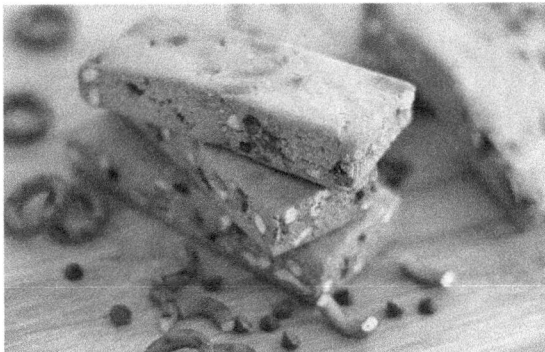

Whenever you are pushed to go for a chocolate bar, which has 225 calories, instead choose to eat a protein bar that normally contains 150 calories. As its name implies, protein bars are very rich in protein. And if you want your protein bar sweet, you can cover it with some chocolate. Try to go for a protein bar that has about 15 grams of protein, 5 grams of fat and not up to 10 grams of carbohydrates.

Berries and Tamari Almond

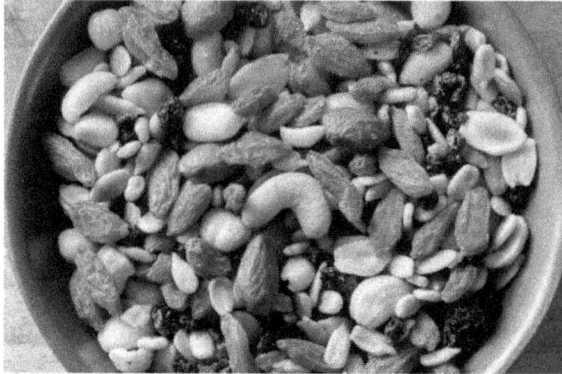

Berries and tamari almond are more nutritious than dried fruits. When you go for a mixture of blueberries, tamari almonds and goji berries, you are improving your health through the production of Human Growth Hormone (HGH).

HGH helps destroy fat in human body and strengthen your muscles. HGH is normally regarded as an anti-ageing agent in human body. So, you should go for a mix of 50 grams of blueberries, 10 grams of goji berries and 10 grams of tamari almonds.

In case you cannot find these types of berries in your locality, do not hesitate to replace them with other berries. All berries have almost the same characteristic composition of dietary fiber and protein.

Natural Yogurt

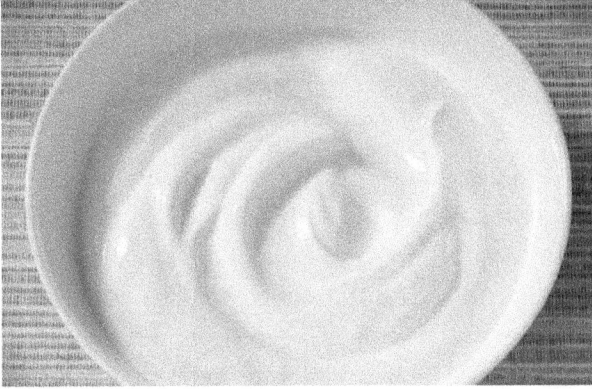

Run away from diet yogurt that contains about 200 calories. Instead, go for the natural yogurt with about 160 calories. You can enjoy your natural yogurt by sprinkling some other nutritious food item on it, for instance, cinnamon. Do you know that 3 to 6 grams of cinnamon per day will produce a significant weight-loss miracle in your body?

Frozen Banana

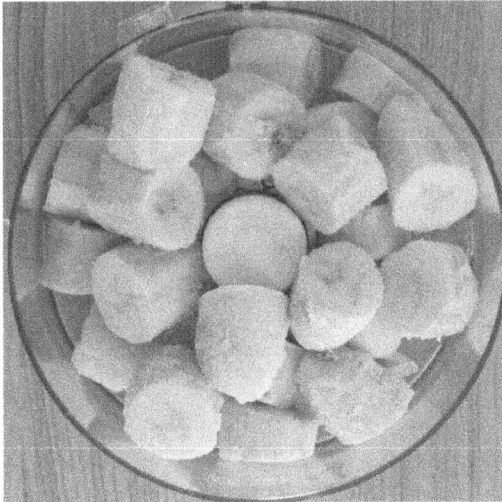

Bananas are highly nutritious and they produce fiber, which is good for losing weight. An average frozen banana has 150 calories, compared with frozen yogurt, which contains 300 calories. One great thing about frozen banana is that it adds no sugar to your body, unlike ice cream. You can mix frozen banana with some natural yogurt and nutmeg.

Do not hesitate to change the ingredients of some of the recommended snack recipes if you find it difficult to lay your hands on them in the area where you live. There are always some other ingredients that produce similar nutrients to your body. If you are unsure about the nature of minerals or nutrients an ingredient contains, do not shy away from asking for some expert advice.

The essence of going on a total body tune up is to emerge victorious at the end shedding two dress sizes. Having the unique opportunity to improve your health through this plan, you should do everything at your disposal to at least make it an outstanding success.

Module 4

Weight Loss Workouts

A great weight-loss plan must consist of two essential parts: The dietary part and the workout regimen. The previous modules have been dedicated entirely to the dietary requirements for losing weight. Now you will be introduced to some of the highly effective weight-loss workouts in human history. Why is it always necessary to do some exercises while losing weight?

Here are three reasons why people are encouraged to workout in addition to their dietary intake during a weight-loss program:

- Workouts increase the rate of your metabolic activities. When you move your body a lot, the motion produces a state of heightened metabolic activities in the organs inside your body.

138

Organic molecules will be quickly digested; increased breathing will allow more oxygen to be inhaled into your respiratory system; moving bowels will confront any problem of indigestion. So, your body system is in a state of hyper-action, and this is very good for your overall health condition.

- Workouts are quite essential for losing weight. When you exercise your body, you are burning some unwanted fat in some parts of your body. Doing an exercise keeps your muscle taut and strong, and it will prevent you from falling sick due to some fat-related illness like obesity and heart problems.

  Think of your body as a piece of machine that needs a regular servicing. And there is no better way to service your body than engaging in a regular and effective workout.

- On top of it all, workouts help people to feel really good about themselves. Regular exercises make you feel light and strong; they improve people's mood and feeling of well-being. Have you ever seen an athletic person who complains a lot about pains in his/her body?

  When you work on your body through regular exercises, you are loosening up all fat molecules stacked in different parts of your body and removing any body and joint pains. People have been advised to work out from time to time in order to maintain the state of well-being they have found themselves through their hard workouts.

These are the three important concerns people often have about working out:

- **When:** Choose a comfortable time-frame and stick to it. You can decide to exercise every morning or evening. And your workout routine could be on weekends when you don't have to go to work or any other engagement. Because human bodies respond to regularity, it is very advisable to choose a specific time and stick to it in for a long period of time.

- **What:** Many people don't necessarily know which types of workouts they need in order to fight some health problems they currently have. This is why it is a good idea to patronize a gym trainer who will help select the list of appropriate workouts you need to combat whatever health concerns you may be having.

- **Where:** Nowadays, you can exercise anywhere: At public or private gym, in your home gym, at the weight management centers, in the municipal sports center and so on. Wherever you choose to go, remember that what is important is not the location but your dedication to benefit a lot from your workout routines.

Don't forget to share your thoughts on this book by leaving a review on Amazon.com. It takes just a few seconds.

Fire Up Your Fat Blasters

Cardio is any exercise, which really gets your heart going. You move about energetically and get out of breath since it is designed to get more oxygen into your blood. When you do cardio, a.k.a. aerobic exercise, your body uses up its fat reserves as the primary fuel source. It therefore makes sense that if you want to get a bikini body, you will need to build in some cardio work.

Here are some top cardio exercises that you can do up to 5 times per week:

1. WALKING

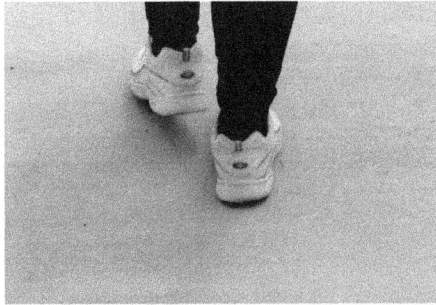

This is ideal for those who are beginning an exercise regime or who are obese as it is low intensity and impacts less on the joints. It typically burns 300-400 calories per hour.

Here's a simple workout. Use a free smartphone app to keep pace:

Walk 3 miles starting on the flat and continue for a mile at a steady pace of 3mph. After the first mile aim to go up and downhill at the same pace until you complete the hour.

2. RUNNING

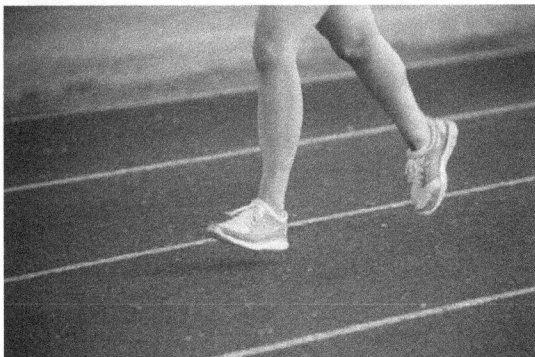

This higher intensity way to lose body fat and improve fitness burns around 600 calories per hour. If you jog (aerobic), rather than sprint (anaerobic), you will burn fat faster. Go for a jog, building your time up to an hour over a period of days, depending on how experienced you are. When you run you also increase your metabolic rate for up to 24 hours afterwards.

3. CYCLING

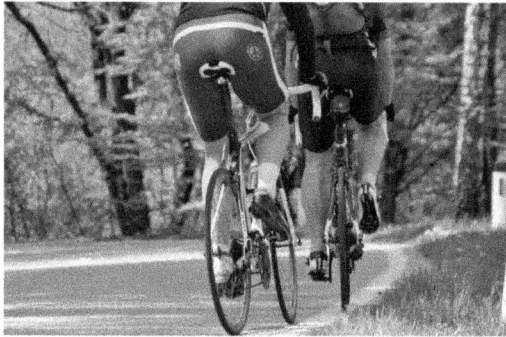

Cycling involves the same muscles as does running, but is a lower impact high intensity way to strip body fat. Use a road bike or stationary bike and be sure to include some hills and inclines.

4. ROWING

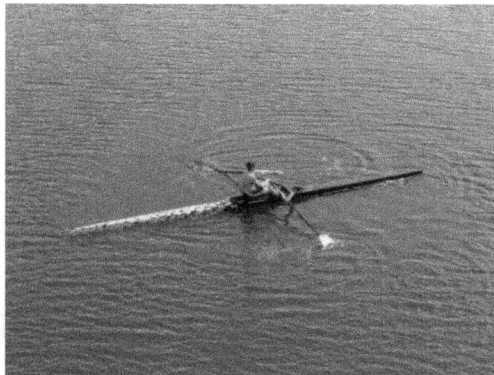

Rowing machines give an excellent total body workout and work the main muscles of the body. Every machine will have its own set of programs and you can burn up to an amazing 840 calories per hour.

5. SWIMMING

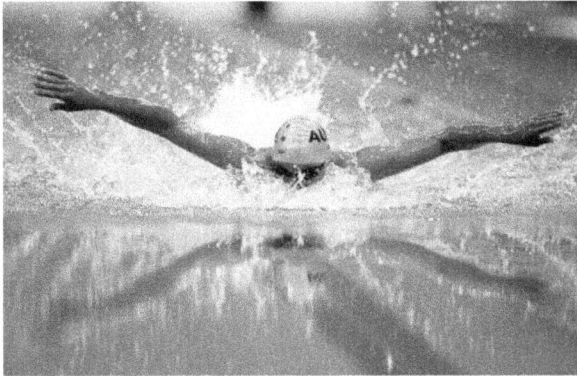

Swimming burns around 600 calories per hour and also provides a great total body workout, while being very low impact and burning a high number of calories.

It will help you burn fat while minimizing the risk of injury. Try this pattern for doing lengths:

- 4 lengths front crawl
- 2 lengths backstroke
- 1 length breaststroke

Rest and repeat for the remaining time, also incorporating butterfly if you can do this stroke.

6. SKIPPING

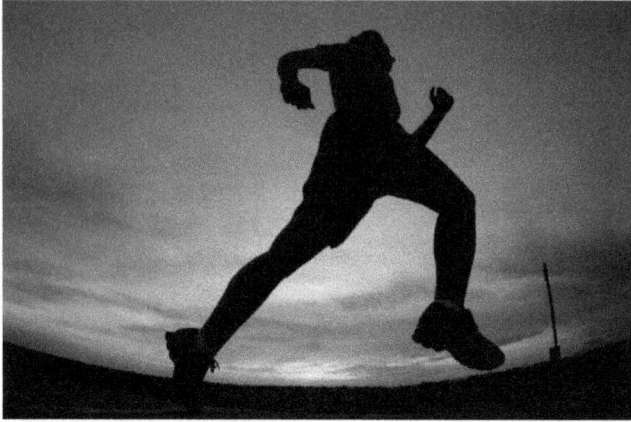

Skipping or jumping rope is a very high impact and hard aerobic exercise. However, the pay-off is that it can be a great fat-burner and it tones, defines and improves strength, speed and bone density too.

Skipping can be quite hard to do, but it you practice your technique it can be a brilliant way to burn calories fast. Just skip on the spot for as long as you can or until the rope gets caught. Try doing 50 skips and then take a minute's rest and start again. Keep going until you are all skipped out!

Try any of the above exercises for up to an hour, 5 times a week, and you will soon see a remarkable difference both on the scales and in the mirror – bikini body here you come!

Total-Body Toning

To make your body firmer and more slender, you will also need some full-body toning exercises. Here are 5 of the best:

Squat and Shoulder Press

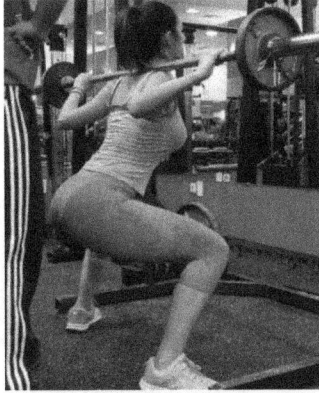

1. Stand with your feet hip-width apart, holding five-pound weights in each hand, with your arms bent and palms facing in.

   Bend your knees and squat, pause, then stand and press your arms straight up over shoulders. Do 10 reps.

Standing Lift

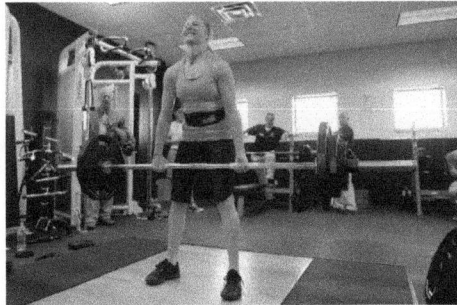

1. Stand with your left foot in front of your right, holding one weight with both hands, your arms extended so the weight is by your right hip.

2. Rotate your arms up and across, pause, then return to start. Do 10 reps, switch sides and repeat.

Side Plank

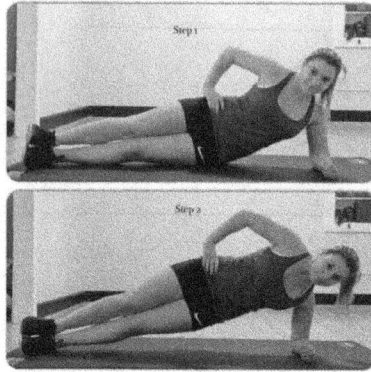

1. Lie on your right side with your legs extended, hips and feet stacked. Prop yourself up on your right forearm, elbow under shoulder, and place your left hand on your waist.

2. Slowly lift your hips off the floor as high as you can. Hold for 15 to 30 seconds then lower to the starting position, switch sides and repeat.

Kickback

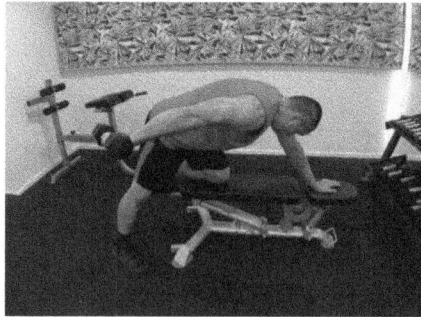

1. Stand with your right foot in front of your left, holding a weight in your left hand. Lean forward with your back flat and bend your left elbow 90 degrees.

2. Slowly extend your arm back, lifting the weight as high as you can and then pause. Lower and repeat for 10 reps, switch sides and repeat.

Inchworm

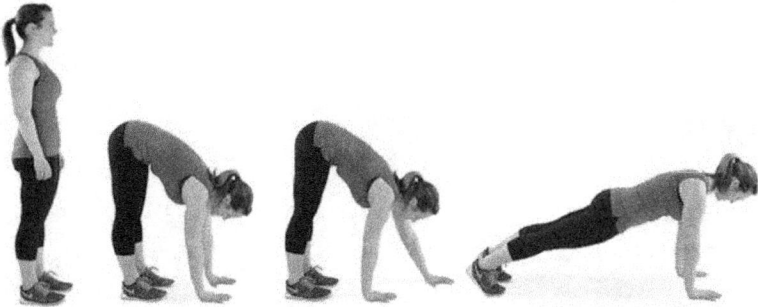

1. Bend forward, place your hands on to floor in front of your feet, and walk your hands forward, until you reach plank position.

2. Do a push-up, and then inch back to the start position. Do 10 reps.

Enjoying this book?

Check out my other best sellers!

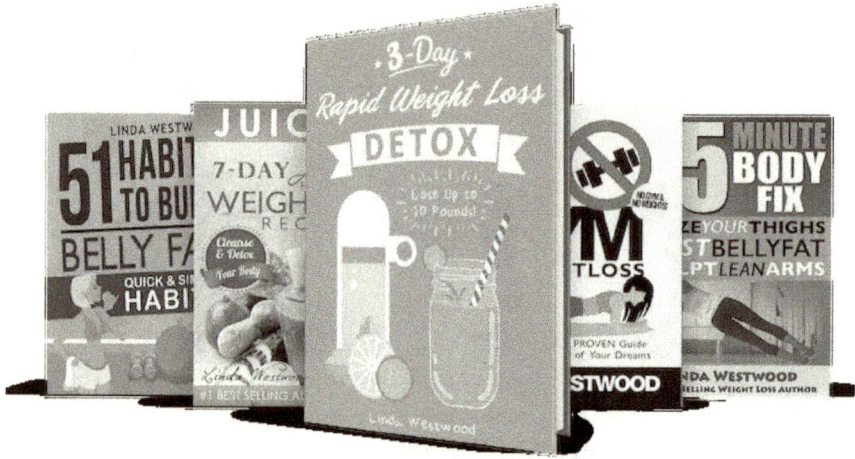

Get your next book on sale here:

TopFitnessAdvice.com/go/books

Cardio Workouts

Cardio workouts are also referred to as cardio vascular trainings. These regimens of exercises are meant to strengthen the muscles around your heart. Cardio workouts are good for increasing your heartbeat rate and for necessitating the in-take of much oxygen. They have been discovered to also help in burning fat, thereby leading to weight loss. However, there are countless theories from different quarters about how best to carry out cardio exercises.

Whatever theories you are subscribing to, here are some eye-opening facts you should always play at the back of your mind while doing cardio workouts. Make sure you do everything you can to avoid these mistakes:

- There is no generalization about how best to do these exercises. Some people believe that having a long cardio exercise over a short period of time is much more effective than doing short cardio over a long period of time. In other words, some people think that doing cardio intensely for 10 minutes will make them burn more fat than doing it with less intensity for 20 minutes. Be careful about this kind of theory: human bodies are different, do not force yourself into doing an intense workout and lose your breath and collapse at the gym. Do what is the best for your body.

- Never do a cardio on empty stomach because people are claiming that they get better results without eating before hitting the gym. Be wary of such unsubstantiated claims. More importantly, do not starve yourself or fail to drink water often as you undergo your cardio exercise. Having a bottle of water beside you is the only wise way to liquidate your body during their energy-sapping exercise.

- Do not follow the crowd to drink energy drink or eat energy food shortly before hitting the gym. Some people believe that last-minute energy drink will make the fat in their body burn more quickly. This is another of those unsubstantiated claims. Or else, you will end up spending your entire exercise time burning the fat you just created through the energy drink or food you had gobbled down!

- Entering your weight and height incorrectly into the machine at the gym. This will give you wrong results at the end of the exercise.

Here are five powerful cardio workouts that can transform your body and burn away unneeded fat in different parts of your body:

Diver's Push-up: Look for a good and spacious place to do this exercise. Start the exercise in a dog-down position. Put your arms firmly on the ground and stare at the floor. In a regular rhythm, move your hips towards the floor as your chest rises. Stay in this motion until your back arched downward and your face is turned to the ceiling. Continue in this fashion for 10-15 minutes.

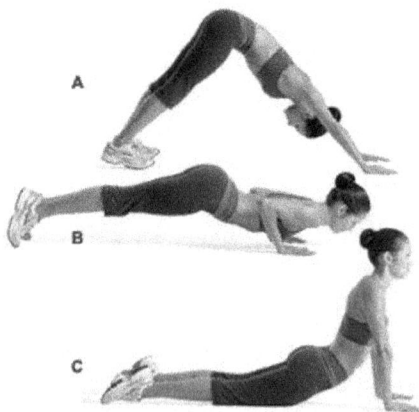

Squat Jump: Do a normal bodyweight squat by keeping your heels on the ground as you bend your knees and hips until your thighs are parallel to the floor. Rise up quickly at the end of the squat and extend your arms overhead. Do this for like 10 to 15 times.

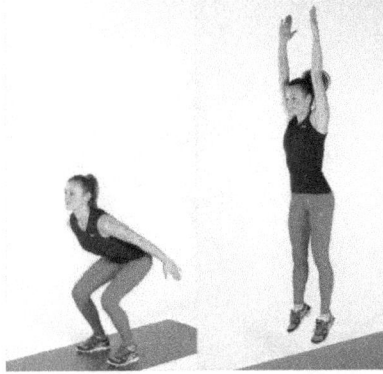

Skater's Lunge: Start this exercise with your legs a bit wider apart, your toes pointing forward. Lower your body into an athletic position, slide to the left into a side lunge while putting your hand on your left knee. Then quickly do the same to your right side. Keep doing this exercise for 50-60 seconds. It should appear as if you are skating on ice.

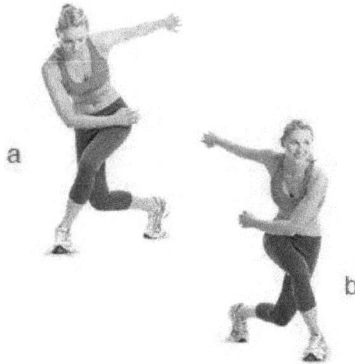

Power Punch: Get ready to behave like a boxer in a training session. Stand with your feet wide apart, putting the right leg in front of the left one. Raise up your fists while your elbows stay in. Punch the air in the front of you, closer to your body while continuously twisting your torso. Punch for like 10 times before changing the positions of your leg and arms (fists).

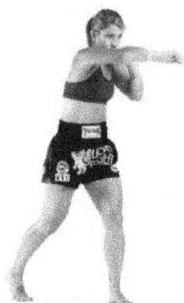

Flutter Kick: You will be doing a lot of kicks in this exercise. Find a good place to lie down on your back. Keep your feet slightly extended while leaving your arms at your sides. Then keep kicking your legs up and down. Do this for about 2 minutes before alternately changing the positions of your arms—which you could keep beside you or hold the back of your head.

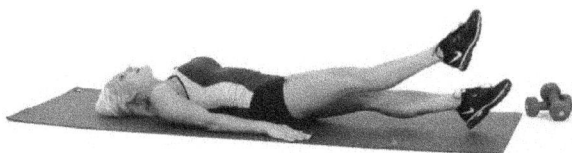

Do not forget to get yourself enough space to these workouts. As you may have noticed, the five exercises highlighted above will affect the fat in your chest, back, legs, arms and neck. If you can successfully burn the fat in these parts of your body, you are well on the way to achieve your purpose—which is to enjoy a total body tone up once starting this weight-loss plan.

Resistance Training

Metabolic resistance training programs are very popular among both men and women. This is due to its unique power to transform human body within a short period of time if done properly. But to make success of it, you must approach it with some determination. Here are the important preparations you have got to make before you can reap any benefits from your metabolic resistance training:

- Define your resistance training goal. That is, which body parts are you targeting to burn their fat?

- Set a time-frame to accomplish this goal. Maybe you are looking at undertaking the training for one month or more. There is no definite time schedule for any of the training. It all depends on your availability and willingness to put in all it takes.

- Find your motivational source: what is it that will be motivating you every day to wake up to do the trainings. We all know it is not always easy to head for the gym and push ourselves through those rigorous exercises.

  So, find a buddy to workout with. Or hire a gym trainer that will keep you focused on it. On top of everything, remember that the exercise is for you—it is for the transformation of your body and not of someone else.

- Don't be too rigid, make sure you adjust your exercise routines as your plan changes. If you have obtained some good results in one area of your exercises, say you have successfully burnt the fat in your arm or waist, change your goal to accommodate exercising some other parts of your body.

- Get a good space for your exercises and use the best equipment out there. Do not harm yourself while using old or out-of-fashion machines. If you are lucky to be patronizing a gym filled up with the latest fitness equipment, use them. If you can't understand how they work, ask for help. It is better to use them successfully and get great results than messing up the whole processes.

So, outlined below are five highly efficient metabolic resistance trainings you can do in the comfort of your home or at a rented gym:

Curtsy Lunge: This exercise helps you work on your hips, abs, quadriceps and hamstring. Be in a standing position with your feel wide apart, putting your hands on your hips. Move your left foot back diagonally and cross it behind the right one. Bend your knees, as if curtsying, as you stretch your left hand towards the floor on the exact outside of your right foot. Go back to the starting position, and do this for 15 times. You can then switch sides (the positions of your feet) and do it repeatedly.

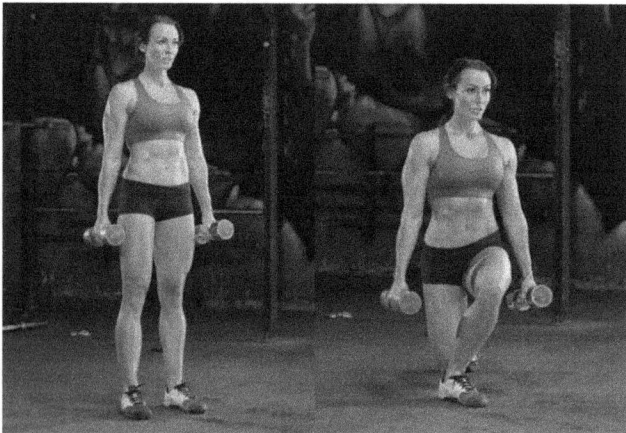

Dolphin Plank: You will be burning the fat in your back, abs and shoulders while doing the "Dolphin Plank". You should lie face down with your toes tucked. Let your forearms rest on the floor. Pull in your bellybutton towards your spine. Then raise your hips to

154

approach the low plank position. You should inhale as you further raise your hips until it forms an inverted V. Pause, then return the starting position. Do this exercise for like 15 times each session.

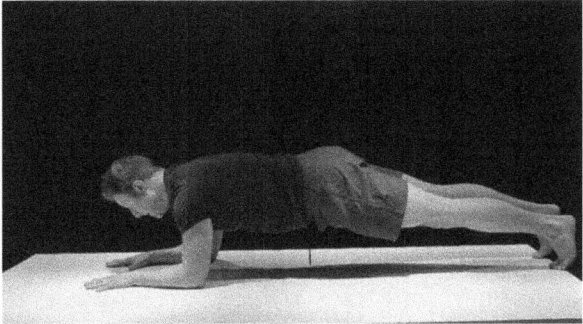

Step-up with Bicep Curl: This is a good exercise for working on the fat in your quadriceps, hamstrings, butt, abs and biceps. You need to stand with your left foot on a sturdy bench or step. Put 5-pound weight in each of your hand. With your weight shifted to your left foot, raise it up and let it stand on the step, your right thigh is also lifted so that it is parallel to the floor. At the same time, lift up each of the weight in your hand to your shoulders, one at a time. Go back to the starting position and repeat the same processes for 15 times.

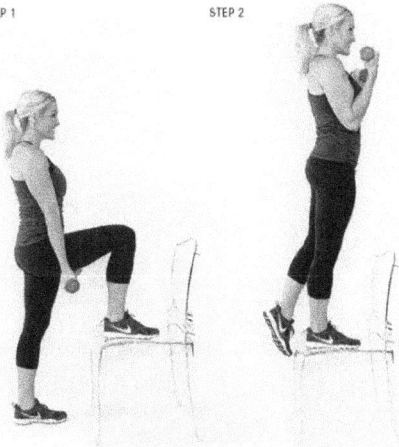

STEP 1   STEP 2

155

Single-Leg Dumbbell Roll: If you are planning to burn the fat in your back, shoulders, biceps, abs, quadriceps, hamstrings and butt. Be in a standing position while holding a 5-to10-pound weight in your left hand. Lunge forward so that your back is flat and almost in a parallel position to the floor. Let your right hand rest on a chair or shelve for support. You should extend your left arm towards the floor so that your palm is facing in.

Raise your left leg behind you so that your body perfectly forms a T-position. Then slowly bend your left elbow and pull your weight up so that the elbow is even with your torso. Hold yourself in that position for a moment and then lower your body (weight) again. Do this exercise for about 15 times; don't forget to switch the positions of your legs, arms and elbows.

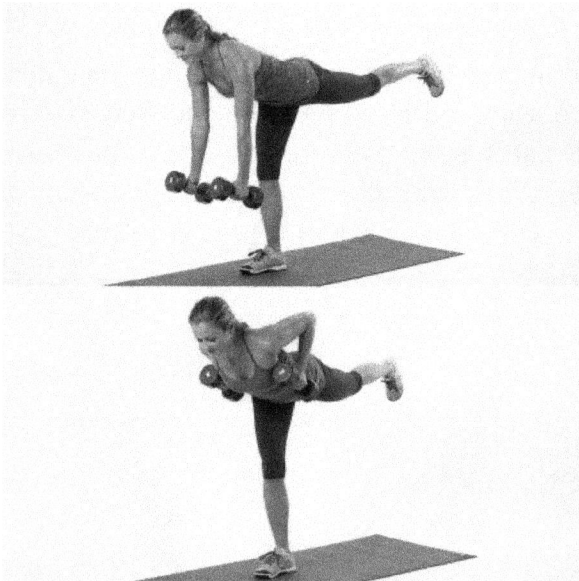

Squat to Overhead Press: Use this exercise to remove the fat in your quadriceps, hamstrings, butt, abs and shoulders. Start by standing with your feet slightly apart. Bend your elbows while holding 5-pound weight in each hand, raised at shoulder height, with palms facing forward. Gently lower your body into a squat, but do not let it go too low close to your toes. Use your heels to push up your body, lifting weights overhead. Then go back to the starting position and do this unique exercise for 15 times.

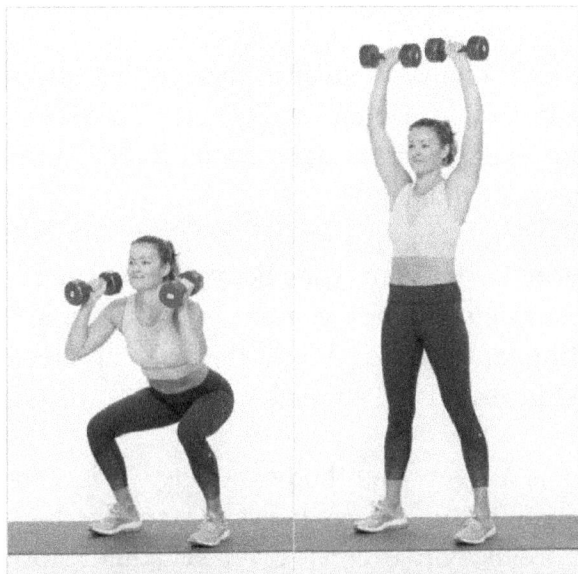

Fast-Track Your New, Sexy Body

The best way to boost your metabolism is through exercise. Not only does cardio boost your metabolism during the workout, but stays elevated for up to 6 hours after the workout is over. It is also important in helping you to deal with daily stresses.

Ideally you should be getting in at least a half an hour's worth of cardio daily. Recent research suggests that it is not even necessary for this to be all at once, as long as you get the required 30 minutes in total every day.

Considering the metabolism boosting effects, it does make sense to split the cardio up into two sessions daily. You do need to be careful not to exercise too close to bedtime as this will result in you not being able to get to sleep. Make sure that you finish your last workout at least four hours before bedtime.

Start the Day the Right Way

Always do at least one workout just after getting out of bed, before you eat your breakfast. Doing cardio before breakfast forces your body to use any existing stores of fat rather than just using the easily accessible energy in your meal.

Contrary to popular wisdom, your body does not need to be fueled before a workout and, unless you are going to do a really intense workout lasting at least an hour, there is no need to take in electrolytes while exercising either.

All you need is to get your body moving. This gets your blood pumping and you get an energy boost to start the day off with. You are also far more likely to exercise if you schedule it for earlier in the day – if you get at least one session over and done with, there is less likely to be anything that will get in the way of your session.

What Exercise do I do?

Initially, this is going to depend on how fit you are at the moment. I know that when I started to exercise, I could not have run down the road, not to mention around the block.

I also had a few false starts when it came to exercise – I tend to be extremely motivated when I start doing things and fade out a little as my motivation wanes. I would really give it my best for the first few sessions then, usually after about a week or so, I'd be feeling sore and tired and just not interested in carrying on.

Once I figured out what the problem was, I managed to get over that. The key to maintaining motivation is to implement small, mini-goals and work towards achieving those and this is doubly true when it comes to exercise. If you have been a couch potato for the last 10 years, you cannot expect your body to take too kindly to working out daily for an hour. And your brain will side with your body on this issue – overdoing the exercising in the early stages will sap your energy and you will find it harder and harder to keep it up.

What you may be surprised to find out though is how quickly your body gets used to the extra exercise once you get into a routine. Initially, your mind will tell you that the body cannot handle this extra activity but once your body starts getting used to being jolted out of its comfort zone, you will find that you actually start to look forward to your exercise sessions.

Okay, this surprised me as well but it does make senses – we were not meant to sit on our butts all day. I know that you really, really want to get going with exercising but I do caution you to take it slowly, at least at first. Rather start off slowly and enjoy progressing to increased levels of fitness than overdoing it completely and quitting altogether.

This also makes the transition less painful. I am not going to lie to you, you are going to find out about muscles that you never knew where there and this will be a bit of a painful exercise at first. You can expect to feel as though you have a mild form of flu for the first week or two, while your body gets accustomed to the increased activity. This is a good sign – it means that what you are doing is having an effect.

Just keep in mind that the "No pain, no gain" mantra of the '80s has since been disproven. While a little discomfort is normal, you should not push your body to the point of pain while working out. What you can do is to schedule a few massages for yourself. A good sports massage will help loosen up painful muscles and will help to reduce the buildup of lactic acid in the muscles. You can also soak in a warm bath at the end of the day. Throw in a cup or two of Epsom salts to help relieve the ache.

Alternatively, get yourself an ointment to rub into your muscles. Ibuprofen can help if you are really, really sore. If you are really battling with pain to the point of needing an analgesic, you need to slow down. If you have led a fairly sedentary lifestyle, I would advise you to have a check-up before starting to exercise. I would not advise you to join a gym, at least, not yet. A gym can be intimidating for you if you haven't exercised for a while. What you need to do is to make it as easy as possible for you to exercise every day until you get into the habit and start to enjoy the exercise.

In one of my failed attempts at exercise, I joined the gym with my brother – BIG mistake because he was a fitness freak at that stage. He had lost quite a bit of weight himself and had done it by pushing and pushing himself. When we got to the gym, he decided it was his job to motivate me. He worked out for at least an hour so I was to do the same. What he didn't take into account was that I was nowhere near as fit as he was. Gym became a nightmare for me – he and I would do cardio together and I could never keep up. I started to loathe the very idea of going to the gym.

Then, to top it all off, he insisted on an hour's exercise and about half an hour in the steam room. By the time you figured in the time it took to get changed, etc. we were spending at least two hours at the gym every night. When he decided that we were to go in the early morning instead, I gave up and never went to that gym again. I had made two mistakes there – I had chosen the wrong exercise buddy and I lost 2 hours out of my day.

Consider Swimming

Swimming can be a gentler way to ease yourself into exercising on a regular basis. The water supports your weight and provides resistance at the same time. It is also a fairly simple exercise and requires little specialist equipment. It does pay to find an Olympic size swimming pool and, if it is cold where you are, a heated one. Most of the bigger gyms do have indoor swimming pools. Swimming is great for overall toning of your muscles and getting you a bit fitter but it is not going to lead to significant weight loss – for that you will need to look at doing more cardio. A couple of colleagues and I once signed up to swim in a mile-long race.

We trained almost every day for two months and, at the end, were able to swim for 60 lengths of the Olympic sized swimming pool without stopping. Training for an event can be great motivation to keep you exercising so have a lookout for events like marathons, etc. over the next few months to consider training for.

Finding the Right Exercise Buddy

An exercise buddy is actually a really good idea – you keep each other accountable for turning up to exercise and motivate each other to continue. You are less likely to miss an exercise session if you have a buddy because you do not want to let them down. Not wanting to let my brother down was one of the reasons that I stuck it out at the gym as long as I did but towards the end I wanted to hit him with a barbell. He, to this day, cannot understand why I got so cross with him and teases me for "not being able to hack it" at the gym.

If I had chosen someone who was more or less at the same level as I was, I would have been better off. We could have progressed together. Reconsider the idea of a buddy if the buddy you choose is a lot fitter than you. Whilst not everyone would be as horrible as my brother was to me, a much fitter person may have forgotten how hard it was in the beginning. Even worse, you might end up feeling that you are holding them back.

Looking back, I should have also found someone who was more supportive. You need to strike a balance between someone who will molly coddle you and someone who will act like a tyrant.

Slowly Slowly Wins the Race

My second mistake was to go from zero to a two-hour commitment so quickly. For me, that was a lot of time, especially since there were things that I would rather have been doing. If you start out with a few minutes a day, it is not much of a commitment in terms of time spent but it is going to be enough for you to see some benefits. If you suddenly have to get up an hour earlier to fit a grueling exercise schedule into your day, you are not likely to maintain it for very long at all. Make it easy on yourself until you get into the habit of exercising every day – I cannot emphasize that enough. It was when I realized this that I actually finally managed to start an exercise program that I stuck to. And it was easy, at first – I walked to the post box and back. That's it – no special equipment needed and hardly any effort either.

Physically, it probably didn't do me all that much good but mentally it was working for me. I was finally getting off my butt and doing something to make my life healthier and it felt pretty good. Before long, I added a circuit around the garden as well. As time went on, I built on that. Eventually I migrated to taking the dogs for daily walks – I now walk 4-5 miles a day. I could even jog if I really wanted to but I am not a fan of jogging.

What I do in order is to change up the route and to include hills so that the route becomes harder. I also alternate between walking slowly for a minute or two and then speeding it up for about three minutes. This is known as interval training and it has been proven to be more effective at getting you fit than exercising at the same pace throughout – even if that pace is the faster one.

Walking is a Great Exercise

I remember Oprah running a campaign a few years ago to get everyone to walk ten thousand steps a day. According to the experts, that was the minimum requirement to keep healthy. I rushed out at once and bought a pedometer and I found that this motivated me to walk for longer distances. For me it was a gimmick but it was a gimmick that worked.

If you find something that works to motivate you to exercise, go ahead and get it. A heart rate monitor is something that can be very useful. You should not let finding the right gimmick make you put off exercising though. There is a fine line between planning an effective schedule and collecting the right tools and wasting time.

Get started today. You can plan your full schedule later on but start walking TODAY. Walking is free, it requires no special equipment. (Though it is advisable to step out of your stilettos and into a more comfortable shoe). Walking is a simple exercise to incorporate into your life. The point is that there really is no excuse not to exercise. You must start moving. Commit to some sort of exercise right now. There really is no excuse for you not to.

You Have to Love it

What made walking so effective in my case was that it was something that I enjoyed, it was something that fitted into my life easily and I finally found the right exercise buddies – the dogs. (Dogs are great companions as exercise buddies – they never moan at you and always love to go for a walk.)

Since then I have tried other forms of exercise as well – some I adopted, some fell by the wayside. I tried Tae Bo, as one example, and found that I lacked the co-ordination to continue with it. I then found an exercise tape that was based on Latin dancing and I loved it. Find out what you love! When it comes to exercise it's going to be a case of trial and error – I tried Pilates and I tried Aerobics and I wasn't that impressed. The Latin dancing and yoga I still do to this day...

Find something that you enjoy – be prepared to try out different types of exercises. Most people think of aerobics classes when they think of cardio but all cardio means is that you are strengthening your cardiovascular system. Anything that gets your heart rate up can be considered cardio.

Can Cardio Help Me Burn Fat?

Cardio will help you to improve your fitness levels and use more energy so, yes; it will help you to burn fat as well. To maximize your fat burning potential during cardio, you are going to need to monitor your heart rate. Now, surprisingly enough, exercising as hard as you can manage is not the best way to lose fat.

It is a better way to get fit but if you want to lose fat, you are going to need to exercise at a level that raises your heartbeat to no more than 80% of maximum. You actually have a reason to slack off a bit when it comes to exercise – isn't that great?

How to Work Out What Your Maximum Heart Rate Is

This is actually fairly easy. You just take your age and subtract it from 220. That is you're approximate maximum heart rate. If you don't have a heart rate monitor, you can simply gauge how hard you have been exercising by your ability to carry a conversation. If you are puffing hard and cannot talk to someone while you are exercising, you need to slow down a little.

Be Consistent

When it comes to cardio, consistency is more important overall than the amount of time you spend on it. Exercising for 10 minutes daily is better than two one hour sessions a week, for example, even though you are not spending as much time on it.

There are going to be days when the last thing that you feel like doing is to exercise. On these days, make a bit of a compromise with yourself – just exercise for 2 minutes and see how it goes from there. 9 out of 10 times, it is getting started that is the hard part and you will find yourself completing a full workout anyway.

Strengthen Your Weak Points

Now that you have a bit of background on exercising, we are going to look at areas that you want to work on specifically. Check out your body and select the areas that you would most like to improve. Note – we do not hate any bit of our bodies; we just have areas that we would like to improve upon.

Take a look at your body and determine what areas you want to give the most attention. Maybe you want to focus on your abs, your thighs or maybe your whole body. Choose a spot and focus on it. Whilst spot training cannot be effective on its own, it can help to whittle down areas that you have a problem with.

Whilst I wanted to lose weight overall, it was my arms and stomach that I really battled with. I never felt confident wearing sleeveless tops because my arms were so flabby so I made a point of researching what types of exercises were best suited to flabby arms and made sure that I included plenty of these in my workouts.

In the next few chapters, I am going to give you tips on dealing with the 5 areas that women most commonly want to work on – the waist, the thighs, the butt, the arms and the chest. I will deal with how to go about toning and strengthening each of these muscle sets in particular so that you can choose which is most important to you and work on that area.

Simply choose the set of exercises pertinent to the areas that you want to improve and schedule sessions three times a week, leaving a day in between each workout for your body to recover. You can schedule these exercises straight after your cardio session if you like. As with the cardio exercises, it is best to schedule the sessions for earlier rather than later as this increases the chances that you will complete them. These spot exercises, when combined with the diet and cardio, are very powerful tools when it comes to toning up and looking great. I will also include tips on how to maximize weight loss and muscle tone for each area.

Take a measurement of each "problem" area and make a note of it. Once a week you are going to take measurements so that you can see what your actual progress in each area is. The exercises in the upcoming chapters are for specific target areas. If you are not sure where to start or want to work on your whole body, here is a simple basic strength building routine to get you started.

A Basic Strength Training Regimen

If you really want to reshape your body, you will need to incorporate strength training into your workout. A lot of women are scared that strength training = big muscles, but this really is not the case at all. You don't even need to join a gym to be able to do strength training.

Here is a very simple workout. Read through all the exercises properly to make sure that you understand what the instructions are before moving forward.

How it works: Twice a week, do 1 set of 12 to 15 reps of each move in order, resting 30 to 60 seconds between exercises. After 3 weeks, increase the weight and/or do 2 sets.

You'll need: A stability ball or chair and a pair of 3- to 5-pound dumbbells.

A Simple Squat

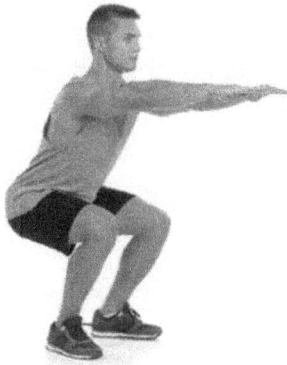

1. Stand with a stability ball between your back and a wall (or tree!), walk feet forward until they're slightly in front of your hips, and place hands on thighs.

2. Squat until thighs are parallel to ground. Rise up onto balls of feet as you reach arms overhead. Return to starting position.

NOTE: You can do this move without a ball—simply press your back against the wall.

Tripod Row

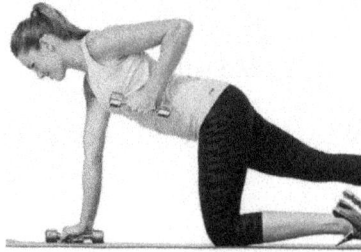

1. Hold a dumbbell in each hand and get on all fours with wrists under shoulders; extend right leg behind you.

2. Bend left elbow, drawing weight toward left side. Lower the weight finish off the rep. Do 12 to 15 reps; switch sides to complete set.

Curl to Press

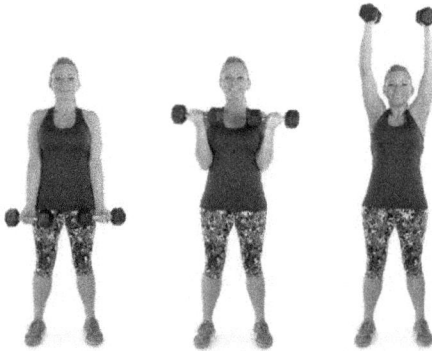

1. Hold a dumbbell in each hand and sit on a stability ball or chair with knees bent and feet on the ground. Extend arms at sides, palms facing forward.

2. Curl weights toward shoulders, and then rotate palms away from you as you press dumbbells straight overhead. Reverse the motion to return to starting position.

Fly to Triceps

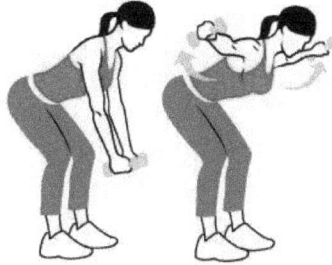

1. Hold a dumbbell in each hand and lie face up with knees bent and heels on a stability ball (press it against a wall for extra stability) or chair. Extend arms over chest, palms facing each other and elbows slightly bent.

2. Lower weights out to side; return to starting position. Then bend elbows, lowering weights toward head. Extend arms back to starting position.

Lying March

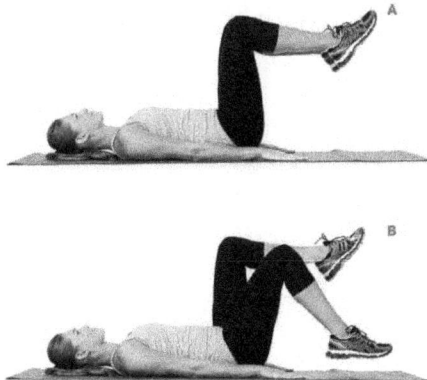

1. Lie face up with knees bent 90 degrees and aligned over hips, arms extended at sides, and palms on the ground. Pull abs in, then slowly lower left foot, stopping just before it touches the ground.

2. Raise left leg to starting position and repeat on right side to complete 1 rep.

Now Stretch

Incorporating a pre- and post-workout stretching routine is important to help properly warm up and cool down muscles when you work out. Stretching lengthens and soothes the muscle tissue, toning it at the same time. It can also assist in speeding away the lactic acid buildup in the muscles. It is the lactic acid, which leads to the muscles feeling sore after exercise.

In general, stretching is important for the good health of your body and should always be considered an important part of the program. You don't even need to do that much – 5 minutes is more than enough to help safeguard against injury and to warm up the muscles. Stretching after a workout is equally important because it helps to ease tight muscles.

Here is a basic stretching routine that you can incorporate on a daily basis.

Forward Bend

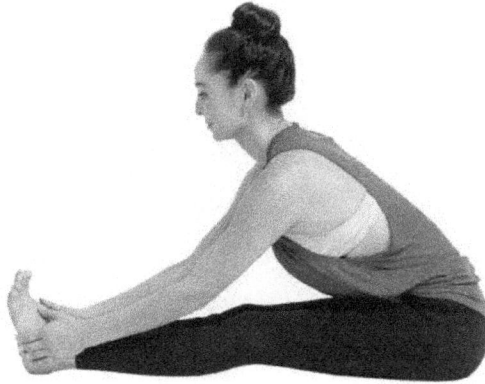

1. Sit on floor with legs extended.

2. Maintain straight back while reaching toward toes (even if you can't touch them); hold.

Runners' Lunge

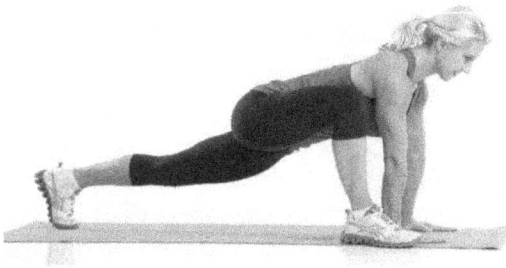

1. Stand 10 inches away from a wall; place palms on it. Step back with right foot.

2. Bend left knee, keeping right heel down; hold. Repeat on opposite side.

Shoulder Stretch

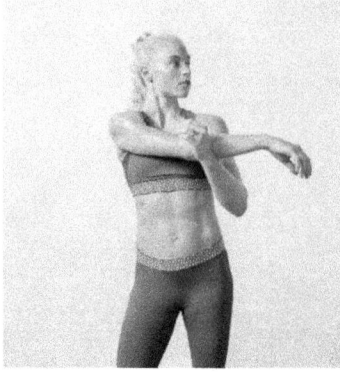

1. Raise right arm and bend elbow over head at a 90-degree angle.

2. Use left hand to grab right elbow and pull it gently to the left; hold. Repeat on opposite side.

Heel Drop

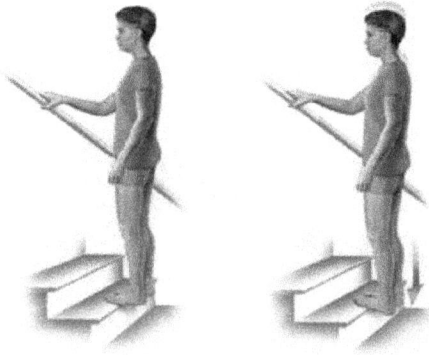

1. Stand on bottom step of a flight of stairs with balls of feet on edge of step.

2. Gently allow heels to drop; hold.

Upward Dog

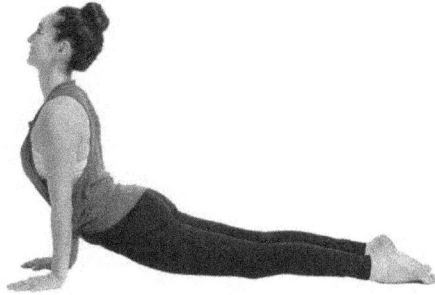

1. Lie flat on your belly. Pushing into your hands, straighten your arms.

2. Lift your thighs off the ground, and keep your toes pointed.

Seated Front-Hip Stretch

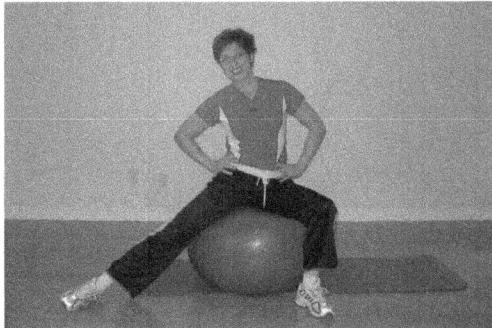

1. Beginning in a sitting position on a fitness ball, straighten your right leg behind you; stabilize by pressing into the floor with the toes on your right foot.

2. Keep your left knee bent and aligned over ankle. Switch sides and repeat. Do 1 stretch on each side.

Tip: To increase the stretch, tuck your hips to roll the ball forward 1–2 inches; hold for 15–30 seconds.

Chest Stretch

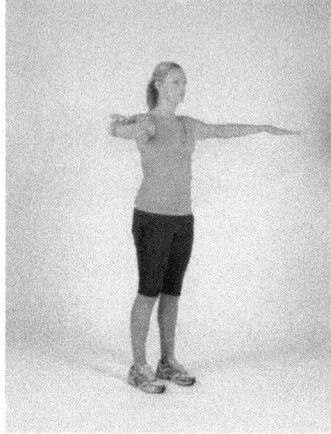

1. Stand up tall, lengthening through the spine. Lift your chest, and relax your shoulders. Look straight ahead, keeping your chin level.

2. Clasp your hands behind your back, and slowly raise arms as far as possible. Hold for 10–15 seconds, breathing naturally.

Knee to Shoulder

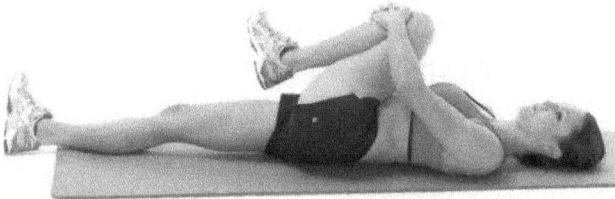

1. Lie on your back with your knees bent, feet on the floor, and arms by your sides. (Your spine should be in neutral alignment with a slight natural curve in the lower back.)

2. Inhale as you clasp your hands around your right thigh; as you exhale, pull right knee toward your shoulder. Hold for 10 seconds.

3. Return to starting position; switch sides and repeat to complete 1 rep. Do 1–3 reps.

Trouble Area #1 – Belly

Many of us find the belly difficult to tone. A lifestyle of over-eating, stress and enjoying alcohol too much can end up laying fatty deposits around the stomach and waist area.

This fat tends to be full of toxins and is particularly bad for our health. Plus too much of it does not look that great in a bikini!

This step will make a big belly a thing of the past with these gut-busting exercises:

Pike and Stretch

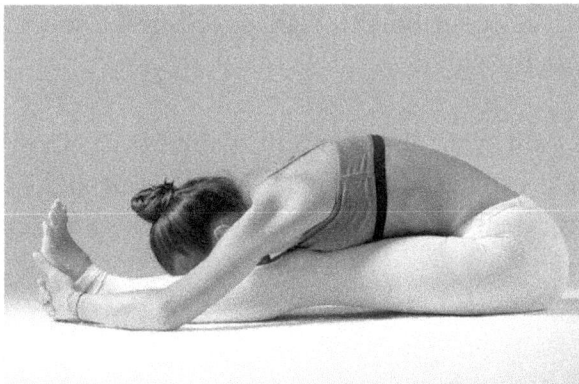

1. Lie face up on the mat with your legs extended over your hips, arms overhead. Crunch up, reaching your hands toward your feet.

2. Keeping your legs straight, bring your arms back overhead as you lower your upper back and your left leg toward floor.

3. Crunch up, lifting your left leg over your hips and reaching hands to feet. Switch legs and repeat for 20 reps, alternating sides.

Standing Side Crunch

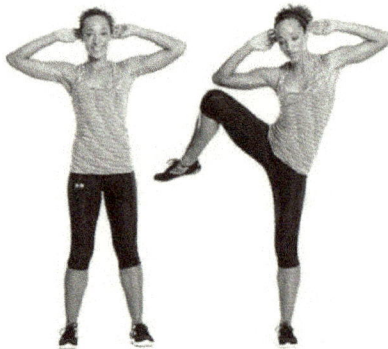

1. Stand on your left leg with your left arm extended out to the side at shoulder height, right foot lifted a few inches off the floor, to the side.

2. Place your right hand behind your head, elbow bent out to the side at shoulder level, then lift your right knee toward your right elbow. Do 15 reps, switch sides and repeat.

Ab-Toning Extensions

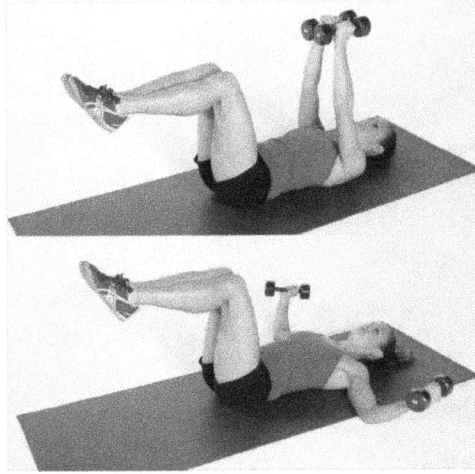

1. Lie face up on a mat, knees bent 90 degrees over hips, holding a dumbbell in each hand, arms extended over chest, palms in.

2. Keeping right knee bent, straighten left leg toward the floor as you lower arms out to sides. Hold for 1 count, then return to start. Do 10 reps, then switch your legs and repeat.

Knee-Up Overhead Press

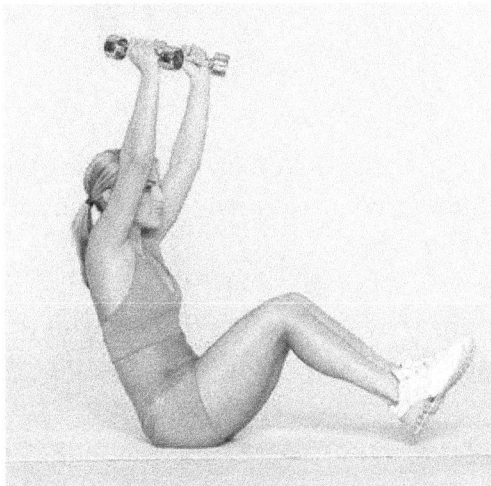

1. Sit on a mat with your knees bent and feet on the floor, holding some dumbbells near your shoulders, elbows by sides, palms in.

2. Lean back slightly and extend your arms overhead as you lift your feet a few inches off the floor and bring your knees toward your chest.

3. Hold position for 1 to 3 counts, and then return to the start. Do 15 reps.

Lunge and Twist

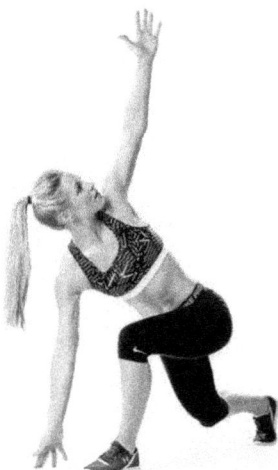

1. Stand with your feet together. Lunge back with your left leg, bending knees 90 degrees, and then reach your left hand to your right foot.

2. Stand up, lift your left knee in front of you to hip height, and bring your fists to your chest, bending your elbows out to the sides as you twist left. Twist to center, lunge left leg back, and repeat. Do 15 reps, switch sides and repeat.

Trouble Area #2 - Thighs

Not many ladies truly love their thighs, but get them into great shape and you will be looking for opportunities to get that bikini back on!

These workouts will tone and trim them brilliantly:

Jumping Squat

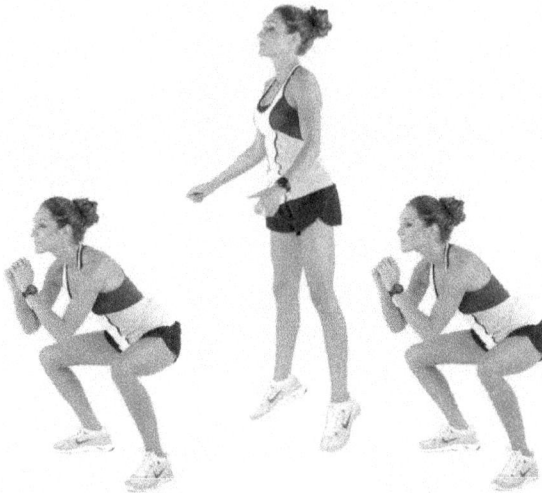

1. Stand with your feet hip-width apart.

2. Squat down, bending your knees to 90 degrees.

3. Now jump up and land softly again in the squat position. Use the strength in your legs and butt to jump up explosively. Remember to land as softly as you can with your knees bent; keep your weight back, over your heels.

4. Do 3 sets of 8 reps.

Leg Circles

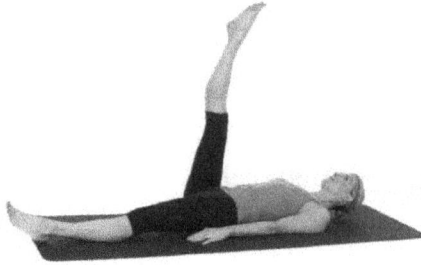

1. Lie back on the mat with your arms by your sides and your palms facing down. Begin by pointing with your left foot, as if reaching out with your toes toward the ceiling, and rotate your leg slightly outward.

2. Inhale, and trace a circle on the ceiling with your left leg, moving your whole leg, but keeping your hips still. Don't lift your left hip off the floor. Trace the circle on the ceiling 5 times in a clockwise direction. Repeat in a counter-clockwise direction. Switch legs and repeat 5 times.

Squat and Lift

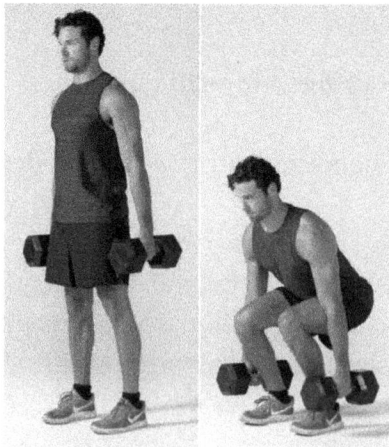

1. Stand with your feet shoulder-width apart, holding a 5- or 8-pound dumbbell in each hand by your sides.

2. Bend your knees 90 degrees, keeping your chest lifted as you place the dumbbells down, outside your feet.

3. Stand up and immediately squat down again, picking up the weights at your feet.

4. Repeat for 1 minute, alternately lowering the weights and picking them up.

Plié

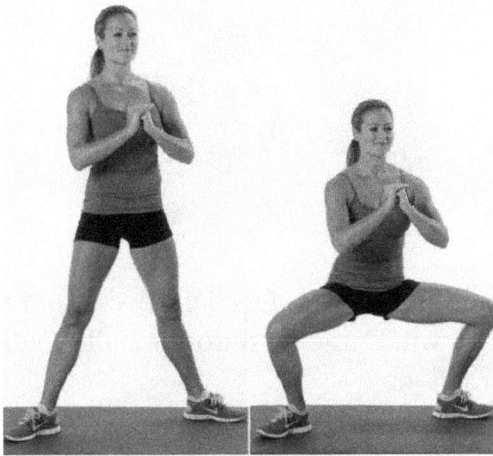

1. Stand with your feet slightly wider than shoulder-width apart and your toes pointing out.

2. Bring your arms out straight in front of you and lower into a squat.

3. Come back up and repeat. Go as low into the squat as you can without letting your knees move past your toes.

4. Be sure to tuck your tailbone under and contract your glutes. Keep your torso upstretched and don't let your knees go past your toes.

5. Do for 1 minute. After about 40 seconds, pulse at the bottom of the squat for 20 seconds.

Thigh Kick Stretch

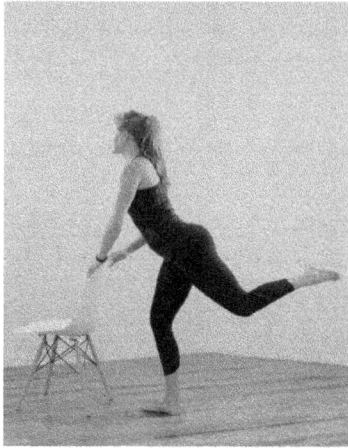

1. Stand holding the back of a chair. Press your shoulder blades back and down. Come up onto the ball of your left foot, and lift your right leg.

2. Keeping your abs pulled in, bring your right leg across your body, in front of your left.

3. Now, swing it back out to the right, keeping your toes flexed and your toes turned out.

4. Do 10 reps. be sure to keep both hips facing forward.

5. Come onto the right leg and repeat for 10 more reps, again making sure your hips are facing forward.

6. Flex your foot as you use momentum to swing your left leg and fire through your right glutes.

7. Rest, then do a second set.

Wide-Stance Squat

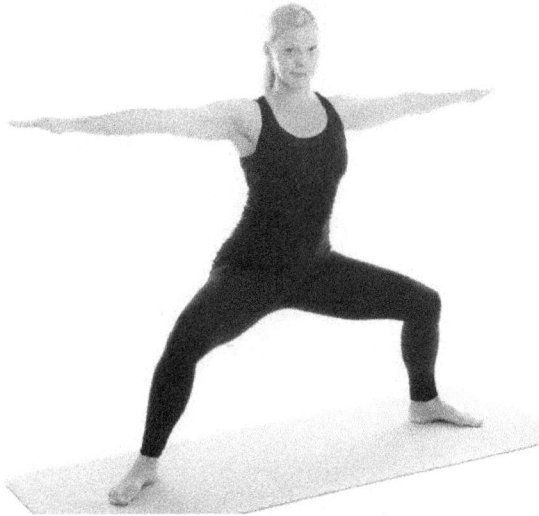

1. Stand with feet slightly wider than shoulder-width apart and toes pointed diagonally outwards.

2. Slowly lower for two counts into a squat position. Hold the squat for one count, then straighten your legs for two counts to go back to the starting position.

Trouble Area #3 - Butt

We all want a tight, toned butt. These exercises are perfect for working out your behind and ensuring you look great from the back as well as the front in your bikini!

Get working those glutes...

Hip Lifts

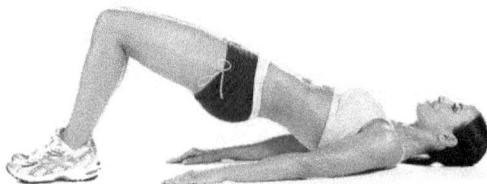

1. Lie on your back with your arms at your sides with your knees bent and your feet on the floor. Lift your hips toward the ceiling. Hold for 1 count, and then lower back down.

2. Repeat the lifts for 60 seconds, squeezing your glutes and hamstrings at the top of the range of motion. Be careful not to overarch your spine.

3. To make this exercise more difficult, extend one leg at the top of the lift. Keep your thighs parallel and hold the lifted position for about 5 seconds.

4. Keeping your hips up, place your foot back on the floor and then lower your hips. Repeat this exercise for 30 seconds; switch sides and do the move for another 30 seconds on the other leg.

Toe Taps

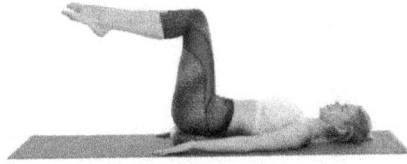

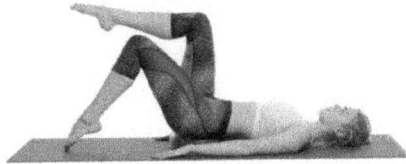

1. Lie on the floor with your arms on your sides. Lift your feet, bending both knees to 90 degrees so your thighs are perpendicular to the floor.

2. Now slowly and quietly tap your left toes to the floor, then your right. Alternate tapping feet for one minute. If you feel any lower back pain, don't bring your toes all the way down.

Dumbbell Squats

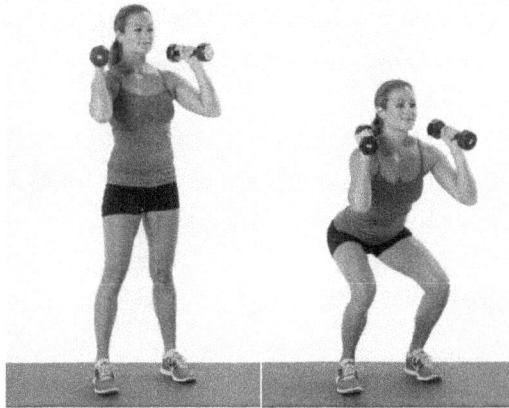

1. Start with your feet shoulder-width apart and 8- to 10-pound dumbbells by your thighs.

2. Squat down as if you were going to sit in a chair, keeping your weight over your heels. Squeeze your glutes as you return to the start position. Do 15-20 reps.

Kick-Back Squat

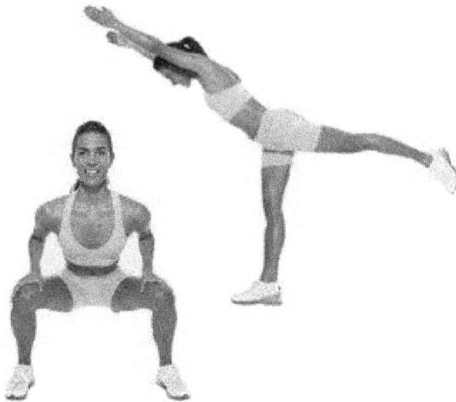

1. Stand with your legs shoulder-width apart. Sit back to a squat, bringing your fists close to your chin.

2. Now bring your left leg straight behind you while extending your arms forward. Return to the squat position, then repeat on the other side.

3. Continue alternating sides for one minute. Keep your weight back on your heels and your hips square.

Super-Lunges

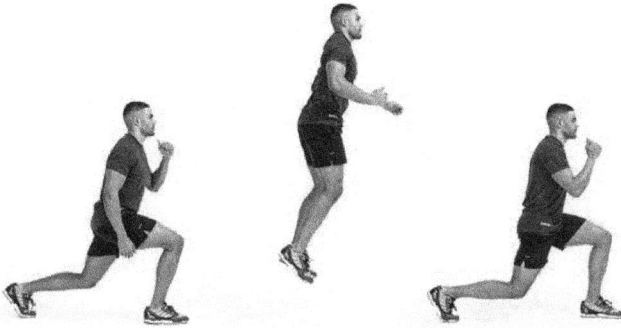

1. Stand with your feet together and your hands on your hips. Then lunge forward with your right leg. Jump up, switch legs in midair, and land with your left leg in a forward lunge.

2. Continue these dynamic lunges, alternating sides, for one minute. Make sure you keep your fists up before your chin and push off the floor with both feet.

Leaning Lifts

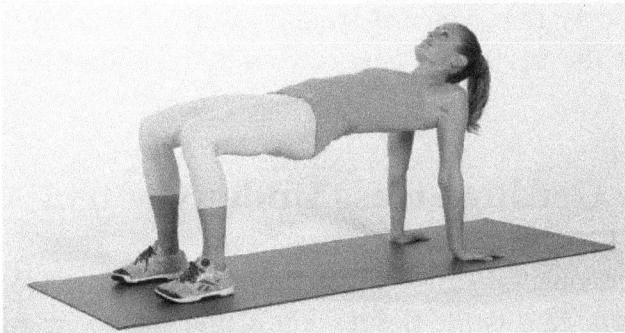

1. Place hands behind the back and tip forward until back is parallel to the floor and flat, abs braced. Take left leg out to the side, resting on toe.

2. Squat with the right leg while simultaneously lifting the left leg a few inches off the ground in a leg lift.

3. Bring the left toe back to the floor and straighten the right leg, repeating for 10 reps before switching sides.

Once again, thank you for reading this book, and I hope you're getting a lot of valuable information. I would greatly appreciate it if you could take 30 seconds to leave me a review for this book on Amazon.com.

Trim Your Waistline & Lose Belly Fat

Belly fat can be deadly. Fat in this region packs on around your organs and begins to increase the number of inflammatory markers in the body. Your risk for developing serious illnesses such as heart disease and diabetes increases substantially. And belly fat is also more difficult to shift. You will find that when you start losing weight, this will be the last place it will move from. Fortunately though, there is a lot that you can do about it.

As a woman, you waistline should measure 80cm or less. For each centimeter over that, you are around about 1 kilogram overweight. Measure at the narrowest part of your waist and write this figure down.

Start by Getting Stress Under Control

Being under constant stress causes the body to release more cortisol. This, in turn, causes the depression of the metabolic rate and an increase in insulin resistance. This, in turn, causes the body to pack on fat in the abdomen area. It is meant as a defense mechanism – during a stressful time, the blood supply to the digestive organs is rerouted so that you are better able to run or fight.

188

The problem with this is that this stress response was only meant to be effected once in a while – not on a permanent basis. And it is not just the physical response to stress that you need to be concerned with – during times of high stress, you are less likely to be able to make healthy choices in terms of what food you eat and are more likely to turn to comfort foods. You need to take steps to manage your stress levels.

Have a look at what you do on a daily basis and identify the stressors in your life as a whole. For most people, stress is a part of daily life, so why is it that some people buckle under the pressure whilst others just seem to coast through? Research has shown that the way you cope with stress is the most important factor when it comes to getting your stress levels down as a whole.

Here are some stress busting tips:

- Socialize – spending quality time with people that we care about is important. You need to have someone that you are able to talk to.

- Exercise – as much as you may not feel physically up to exercising, it is vital that you do. Exercise not only helps to release feel-good hormones but it provides an active outlet for getting rid of the stress hormones as well.

- Me Time – you need some time for yourself to do something that you really enjoy, even if only for 15 minutes or so a day. Me time is not selfish – taking better care of yourself means you are more able to cope properly and everyone benefits from that.

- Laughter is the best medicine – If you are having a really bad day, try pulling out your favorite comedy and watching that.

A good laugh will help to release endorphins and will make you feel a lot better.

- Try yoga, deep breathing exercises or meditation – most of us breathe too shallowly in the first place. If you have time for nothing else, set aside some time every morning and every evening for some deep breathing exercises. Breathe in slowly for a count of 4, hold for a count of 4 and then release to a count of 4.

  Repeat this 10 times and you will feel instantly more relaxed. While doing this, focus on the breathing and try to block out everything else. This in and of itself is a great mini-meditation.

- Switch off – one of the perils of modern living is that we suffer from information overload. Think about it, when was the last time that you were actually unreachable? Thanks to smart phones and tablets, we are practically available 24 hours a day. We also have access to more information than any generation previously and we are becoming more and more stressed as a result. Switch off your phone and laptop for at least a half an hour a day.

- Stop the stimulants – most of us love our cup of coffee in the morning. Many people cannot function without it. That is a sign that something is wrong in your life – if you cannot function without some form of stimulant like coffee or sugar, you need to do a bit of a lifestyle audit.

Exercises to Help You Lose Belly Fat
For Beginners

Lunge Twist

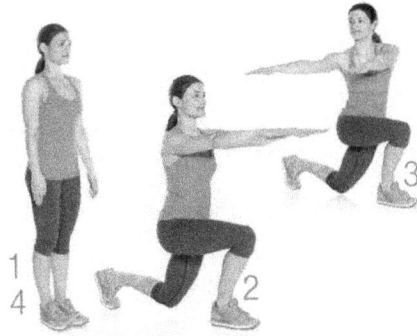

1. Stand with feet hip-width apart, knees slightly bent, elbows bent 90 degrees by hips. Lunge forward with right leg and rotate torso and arms to right.

2. Rotate back to center as you quickly push off right foot to return to start. Do 16 reps, alternating sides.

Step Hop

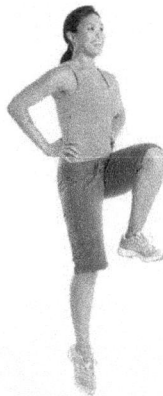

1. Stand with feet hip-width apart, knees slightly bent, hands on hips. Step forward with right foot, then lift left knee to hip level as you hop straight up on right leg.

2. Land with feet together. Do 16 reps, alternating sides.

Shot Put

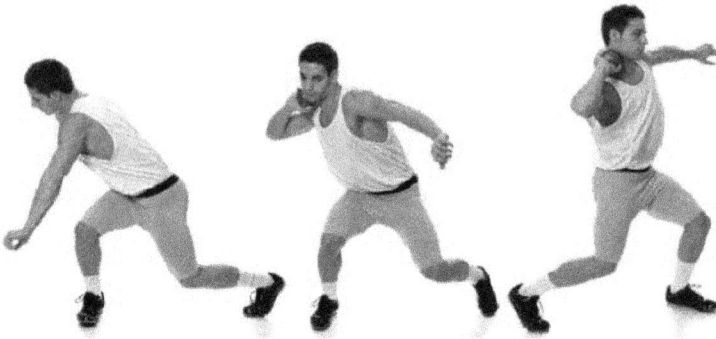

1. Stand with feet hip-width apart, right elbow bent with hand by ear, left arm out at shoulder level. Lunge to right with right leg; rotate torso to right.

2. Push off right foot to stand, pivoting to left. Extend right arm diagonally (as if throwing a shot). Do 16 reps, alternating sides.

Intermediate Exercises

Lunge

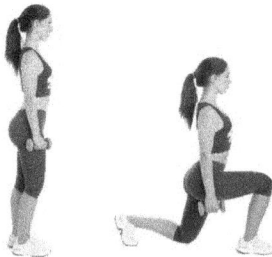

1. Stand with feet hip-width apart, knees slightly bent, arms by sides. Lunge forward with left leg, bending both knees 90 degrees, and reach arms toward floor.

2. Explosively push off left leg to return to starting position and lift arms straight overhead. Do 8 reps. Switch sides; repeat.

Discus Throw

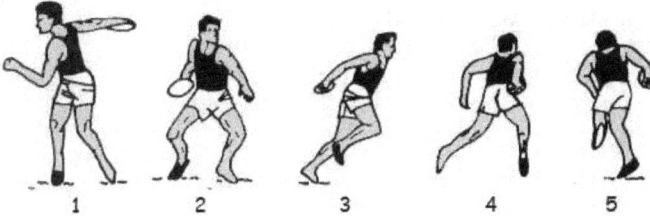

1. Stand with feet shoulder-width apart, arms extended out to sides at shoulder level. Lunge to right with right leg, rotating torso to right.

2. Quickly shift weight to left leg, bend knee, and push off left foot to hop up as you turn to left and swing right arm across body (as if throwing a discus). Do 10 reps. Switch sides; repeat.

Advanced Exercises

Lunge Jumps

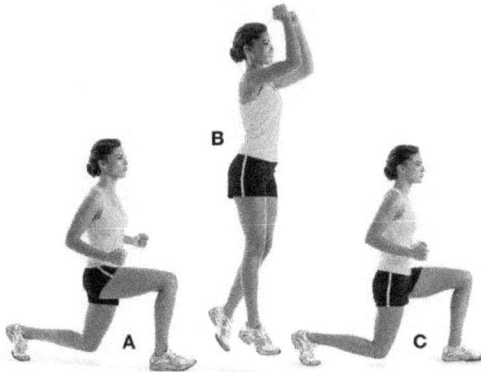

1. Stand with feet hip-width apart, knees slightly bent, arms extended overhead. Lunge forward with left leg, bending both knees 90 degrees.

2. Jump straight up, switching legs in midair, so that you land in a lunge with right leg in front. Do 12 reps, alternating sides.

Squat Jump

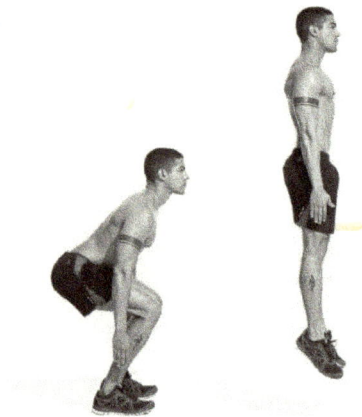

1. Stand with feet shoulder-width apart, knees slightly bent, hands by sides. Squat, keeping knees behind toes, then jump straight up, lifting arms overhead.

2. Land in a squat with arms overhead. Lower arms by sides. Do 12 reps

Hammer Hoist

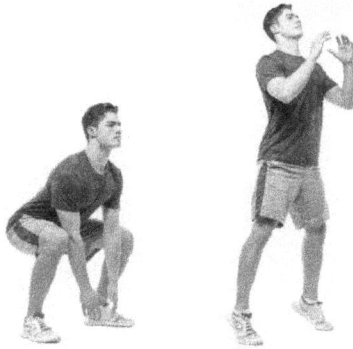

1. Stand with feet slightly more than shoulder-width apart, hands clasped together in front of thighs. Squat, keeping knees behind toes, and reach arms slightly back between legs. Jump straight up, bringing arms overhead (as if hoisting a heavy mallet). Land in starting position. Do 12 reps.

The Crunch – Only Better

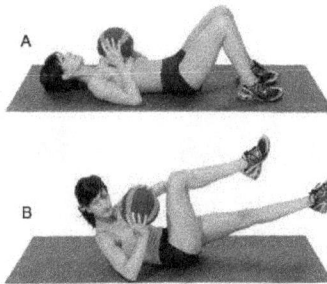

1. Sit so thighs and upper torso form a V shape, with lower legs crossed and lifted. Hold a 5-pound medicine ball (or dumbbell) between both hands. Swivel left to right and back, bringing ball across body while maintaining the V shape. Do 3 sets of 15 reps 3–4 times a week

Simple Arm Reach

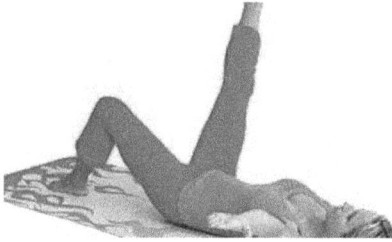

1. Lie face up with your left knee bent, left foot flat on the floor, and right leg extended toward the ceiling. Reach toward the ceiling with your left arm and keep your right arm down by your side.

2. Without moving your hips or shoulders, open your raised leg to the right and raised arm to the left. Now, concentrating on your abs, return your raised leg and arm to the center. Do 10–12 reps, then switch sides and repeat.

Lower Belly Reach

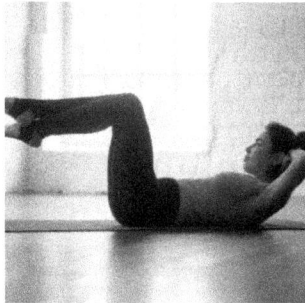

1. Lie face up with knees bent to 90 degrees, hands behind head, and abs contracted. Keeping knees stacked over hips, lift shoulders and crunch up; inhale and hold for 3-5 seconds. Exhale and extend legs to 45 degrees; hold for 3-5 seconds while squeezing lower belly. Do 2 sets of 10-15 reps.

Teaser

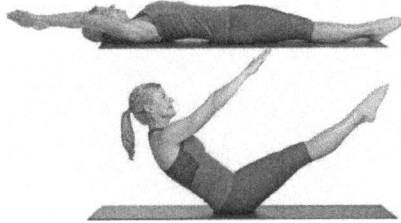

1. Lie on your back with knees bent to 90-degree angles and feet lifted. Tighten abs as you inhale, and lift arms up and back over head.

2. Exhale and swing arms forward, straightening legs so your body forms a V. If needed, put hands on the floor for support. Roll down slowly, bending knees and bringing arms overhead. Do 15 reps.

Donkey Kickbacks

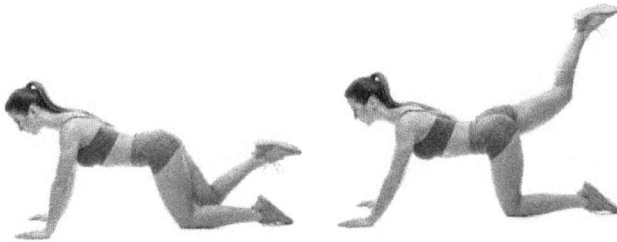

1. Kneel on all fours, toes tucked under, keeping your back neutral. Draw your belly in toward your spine as you contract your abs and lift both knees about 2 inches off the ground.

2. Keeping abs engaged, bring right knee to nose (shown). Then kick right leg straight out behind you, squeezing your butt;

keep lower abs contracted and hips facing the ground to protect your back. Repeat 8 times; switch legs and repeat.

Advanced Leg Crunches

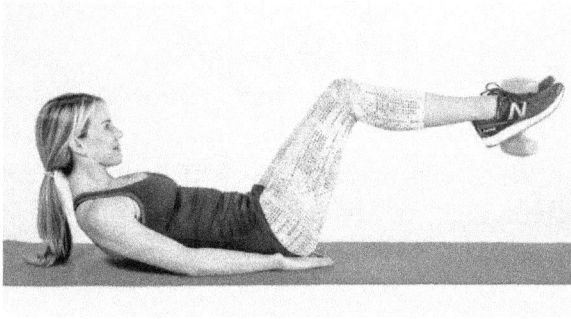

1. Lie on your back with your knees bent and a 3-pound dumbbell between your feet. Place your hands, palms down, beneath your sitting bones.

2. Concentrating on your lower abs, use them to bring your knees in toward your chest while lifting your hips, head, and shoulders slightly. Return to the starting position; that's 1 rep. Do 15–30 reps 3–4 times a week; you should see results in 4 weeks.

Belly Blaster

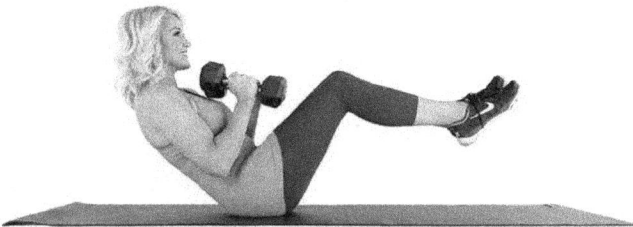

1. Lie on your back with your knees bent in toward your chest. Hold 1 (3-pound) dumbbell with both hands. Extend your

left leg to 45 degrees, keeping your right knee bent. Lift your head and shoulders and move the dumbbell to the outside of your right knee, pressing into a crunch with a twist (shown above).

2. Pull your left leg in to meet your right leg and reach the weight up toward the ceiling, keeping your shoulders and head elevated off the floor. Now repeat step 2, but this time extend your right leg and keep your left knee bent. That's 1 rep. Do 8 reps 4 times per week, and you should see results in 3 weeks.

Scale Pose

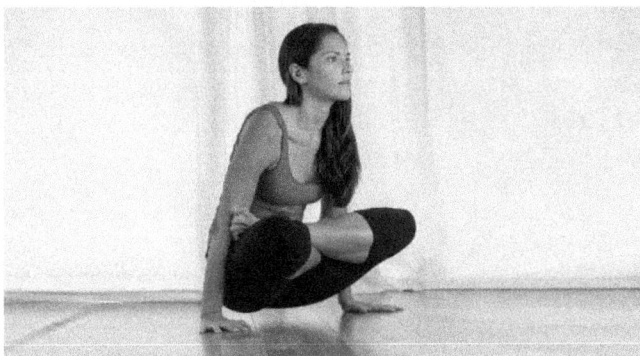

1. Sit in a comfortable cross-legged position with hands on a mat next to your hips. Tighten your pelvic floor (as if you have to pee and are holding it in), push into your hands, and lift your entire lower body off the mat.

2. Hold for 3 breaths and lower yourself. This is an advanced move so if you are not able to lift up your entire body, keep your feet on the floor and just lift your butt. Do 3 reps.

Diagonal Crunch

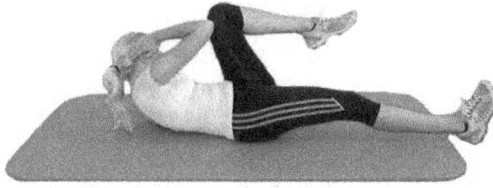

1. Lie on your back with your legs straight and feet on the floor. Keeping your torso still, lift your hips and move them a bit to the right; lower and straighten your legs again.

2. Bend your left knee and cross it over your right leg, placing your left foot on the floor near the outside of your right knee. Crunch up, and then come back down. Work up to 50 reps, then switch sides and repeat.

Toning V-Hold

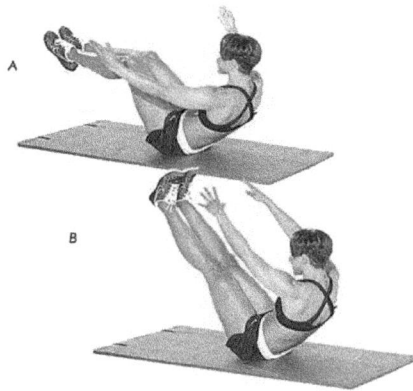

1. Sit with knees bent and feet on floor. Clasp underside of thighs with both hands, hinge back, and lift feet until lower legs are parallel to floor; release hands. Straighten legs and reach for your toes; hold for 8 breaths. Repeat 3 times.

The Plank

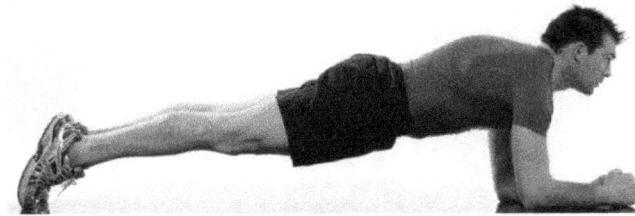

1. Kneel on a mat on all fours with your hands directly under your shoulders. Stretch your legs back one at a time to come into plank position (the "up" part of a push-up); engage your ab muscles.

2. Your body should be long and straight; don't let your hips sag or lift your butt too high. Imagine there's a seat belt tightening around your waist, drawing your lower-ab muscles inward. Press your hands firmly into the mat, and press strongly back through your heels. Hold for 1–2 minutes (or as long as you can), then drop back to all fours. Do 3 reps.

Full Body Squat

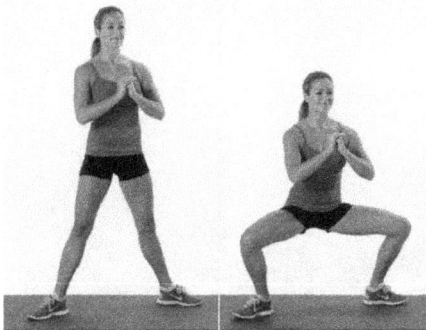

1. Stand with feet hip-width, knees bent slightly, hands crossed over chest. Squat down, pressing weight into feet. Make sure

feet are pointing straight ahead and knees are over your toes; keep bum tucked. Return to standing. Do 8-10 reps.

Windshield Wiper

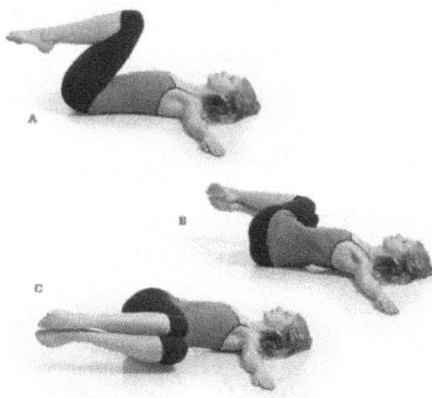

1. Lie on your back with knees bent to 90-degree angles. Straighten your arms by your sides, and lengthen your fingertips. Press the backs of your shoulders against a mat, and slide them down away from your ears.

2. Focusing on the deep waist muscles, inhale and slowly move your knees to the right, then exhale and return to starting position. Repeat on the left; that's 1 rep. Do 5–8 reps.

Plank on the Swiss Ball

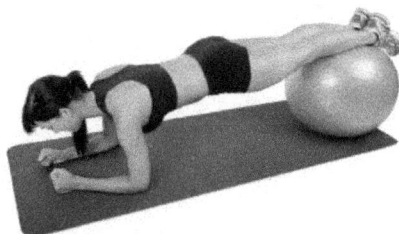

1. Kneel in front of a Swiss ball, draping your abs and hips over the ball. Place your hands on the ground in front of you and walk them out until the ball rolls beneath your thighs.

2. Once your body is straight (with a slight arch in your back) and you're stable, hold for 30 seconds. Focus on lifting belly button and squeezing thighs.

Ball Overhead Crunch

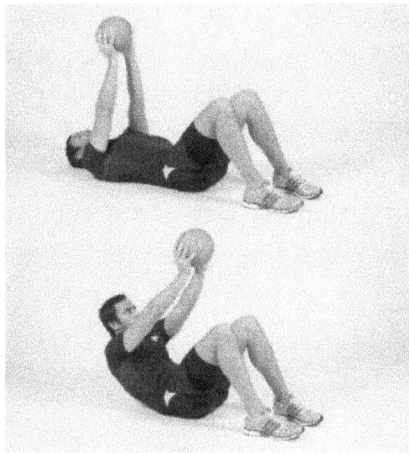

1. Stand holding ball overhead, elbows bent and out to sides, and feet shoulder-width apart. Lift right knee to side; pull right elbow down to meet it.

2. Return to starting position; repeat on other side. Bounce ball for 1 minute. Repeat sequence 3 more times.

Jumping Jack Revamped

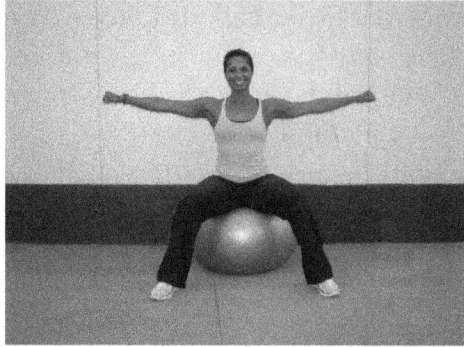

1. While seated, hold the ball and jump legs apart, then together, and then apart again. Stand and reach left hand to the right (use right hand to keep ball in place).

2. Sit back down, jump legs together, and repeat sequence on the other side; that's 1 rep. Do 4 reps, and then do Basic Bounce for 1 minute. Repeat sequence 3 more times.

Everyday Tips to Getting a Trimmer Waistline

Strengthen Your Core

You'll get more from your Pilates, yoga, or core-focused moves—meaning a slimmer, flatter belly—by following these tips:

Move from your waist. Whenever you twist, make sure the movement happens from your bottom rib up. Keep hips still.

Tighten up. Throughout each move, you should feel a tightening, similar to zipping up a pair of tight jeans, from one hip bone to the other.

Exhale deeply. To help strengthen your abs and protect your lower back, be sure to exhale thoroughly with every breath.

Spent time finding out the right way to do the exercises – the correct form is especially important when it comes to exercises to flatten your belly.

Posture is Important

Stand up straight, pull your tummy in and tuck your pelvis under – that is what we learned in deportment classes and it is great advice. Adopting good posture automatically makes you look longer and leaner. It helps to align the organs properly, facilitates energy flow and circulation throughout the body and makes you appear more confident.

Not sure if your posture is right? Stand up against a wall and straighten out completely. Pretend that there is a string extending from your head and straightening you out. Not convinced? Okay, pull out the tape measure. Now take your measurement at the widest part of your stomach. Write it down. Now suck your stomach in as hard as you can.

You lost centimeters instantly, didn't you? What we tend to forget is that we have abdominal muscles. If we don't exercise these, they become slack and the gut slumps forward. They are still there; they just are not working as well as they should. If you are only going to adopt one tip from this chapter – this is the most important one – suck in your stomach. At first, you will actively need to remind yourself to do this.

I found that the only way was to write a note for myself and stick it on the front door, to remind me every time I walked out the house. Over time, it became a habit and now it is second-nature.

You should remember that even if you do tone those muscles up, you will still need to follow the diet to get rid of the fat over the top of them.

Eating for Your Belly

If you have stubborn belly fat, it is important to include the following in your diet:

- Leafy green vegetables – these are an important source of magnesium. In a study conducted by the Journal of Nutrition in 2013, it was found that those who got more magnesium had significantly lower levels when it came to fasting blood sugar and insulin levels. High levels of both are indicators of insulin resistance, metabolic syndrome or diabetes. Magnesium is also important in fighting water retention and bloating.

- Make sure that you get enough monounsaturated fats. It may seem strange to encourage you to eat fats but these are healthy and good for you. They help your body to fight off inflammation and rev up your body's fat burning ability overall. They are the most effective foods to use to target belly fat.

- Look into High Intensity interval Training – this is where strength training and cardio are combined. The exercise is more intense but you get results a lot faster. What you do is to combine strength training and cardio.

  This is also called circuit training. You do your normal strength training exercises but instead of resting between each set, you do some high intensity cardio, like running on the spot, for 3 or 4 minutes at a time.

- According to the American Journal of Epidemiology, those women who got less than 5 hours quality sleep a night were around about 32% more prone to significant weight gain over a period of 16 years.

You are also more likely to eat more calories if you have not slept enough – as much as 300 more calories a day. Lack of sleep increases the levels of ghrelin, one of the hunger hormones, in your body and you feel hungrier.

- Cut out the sodas - even the artificially sweetened ones. Sugar is bad for you, we know that. Artificial sweeteners are no better. Studies into the effects of both show that sugar is actually the better of the two.

  When you drink artificial sweeteners, they do not sate your body's craving for sweetness, leading you to crave even more calories. Plain green tea and water are the best drinks when it comes to weight loss.

- Cut the salt – excessive amounts of sodium cause water retention and bloating. The scary thing is that you are probably having too much salt already, even if you never touch table salt. Salt is used extensively in many different processed foods. Combat this by sticking to natural foods and flavor with herbs and spices rather than salt.

- Watch the alcohol intake – if you are going to drink, stick to the occasional glass of wine or clear spirits. Ditch the cocktails, ciders and sugary mixers.

Get Lean Legs & Sexy Thighs

Getting long lean legs and sexy thighs is fortunately a lot easier than losing belly fat. The muscles in your legs respond extremely well to exercise and will tone up quite quickly. Squats and lunges are amongst the best exercises for the lower half of your body and are easy to incorporate in your day.

Do 10 of each as you brush your teeth, or when doing bicep curls and you will soon see a difference. Intensify these exercises by holding the position at the bottom of the movement. If you are battling with a doing a squat, use a chair to help you maintain your balance – just ensure that you do not use it as an aid to pull yourself up. Alternatively, lean back against the wall and then slide into a squat. This is an easier move for beginners.

Rebounding is a great way to exercise without the danger of impact injuries. It is fun and quick to do and you don't need any special equipment. If you are carrying more weight on your thighs and butt, you need to look at working out at a lower intensity for longer. You should aim for cardio sessions at about 45 minutes as the fat in these areas can be harder to lose than belly fat.

Do try to walk or cycle to work if you can manage it – not only will you not have to worry about getting stuck in rush-hour traffic, for every half an hour extra of activity you could burn an extra 500 calories. Done every day that will translate into weight loss of about 3 pounds a month and will contribute to your overall cardio quota. Can't manage that? Park your car further away when using it so that you automatically have to walk further or climb off the bus/ subway a few stops earlier every day.

Climbing stairs is also a great workout for the legs so try to take the stairs wherever possible. If you live in an apartment block, the stairs are a great bonus for you. Build up your workout by increasing the number of times you climb up and down the stairs each day. You can also vary it by sprinting up the stairs or going up two steps at a time for a greater stretch.

When it comes to the gym, weights are not actually the best option for your legs. It is more important to try and work as many of your leg muscles as possible and the best exercise for this is a side lunge. Hitting the stepping machine and treadmill offer the best cardio options. If your daily exercise routine consists of walking or jogging, you should include some sprints in order to boost the overall efficacy of the workout.

A sedentary lifestyle is especially bad on the butt and thighs. Stand up often throughout the day in order to get circulation pumping. Try standing whenever you are on the phone to get into the habit or make a point of getting up every 15 minutes or so. You need to incorporate some stretching routines and some resistance training in your workouts for maximum benefits. Using a resistance band is especially helpful when it comes to legs and thighs.

Stretching is extremely important to avoid injuring yourself. Hit the beach. Walking on beach sand provides a good workout and can be fun as well – it is harder work to walk on the beach than on an even surface. The most important exercise tip of all is to shake it up once in a while – change up the types of exercises that you do so that all the muscles in your lower body get a workout. There are around 200 of them, so get creative.

Skin brushing can be very effective at getting the circulation flowing and the lymph moving. This can help reduce the appearance of acne on the legs. You need to include more protein in your diet if you are doing strength training as this helps to repair the muscle tissue.

Sculpt A Tight Butt

A nice, shapely butt is on the wish list of many women. The butt is one area that you can work on discreetly throughout the day – clench and unclench your gluteus maximus while sitting at your desk or while waiting in line.

Here are some other workout tips – these are suitable for all levels so just vary the number of reps if you are battling to keep up:

Marching Hip Raise

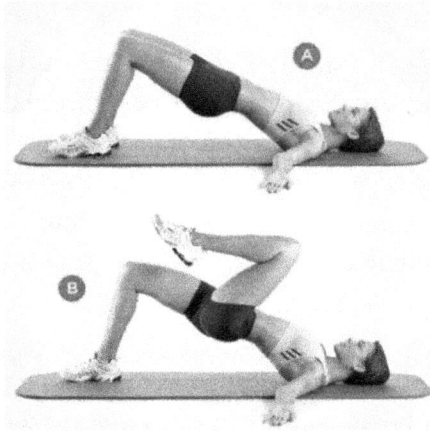

1. Lie face up on the floor with your knees bent and your feet flat on the floor. Raise your hips so your body forms a straight line from your shoulders to your knees.

2. Lift one knee to your chest, lower back to the start, and lift your other knee to your chest. Continue to alternate back and forth doing sets of 8 reps each side.

Single Leg Hip Raise

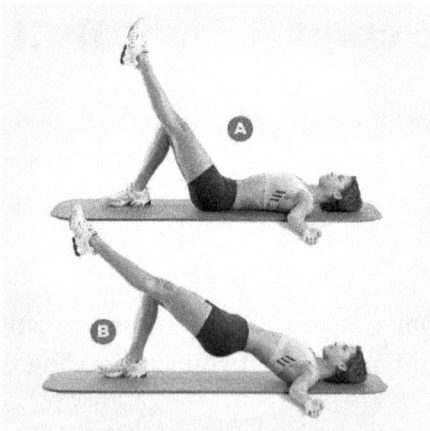

1. Lie face up on the floor with your left knee bent and your right leg straight. Raise your right leg until it's in line with your left thigh.

2. Push your hips upward, keeping your right leg elevated. Pause, and then slowly lower your body and leg back to the start position. Do 8 sets of reps with your left leg, then switch and do the same number with your right leg.

Swiss Ball Hip Raise and Leg Curl

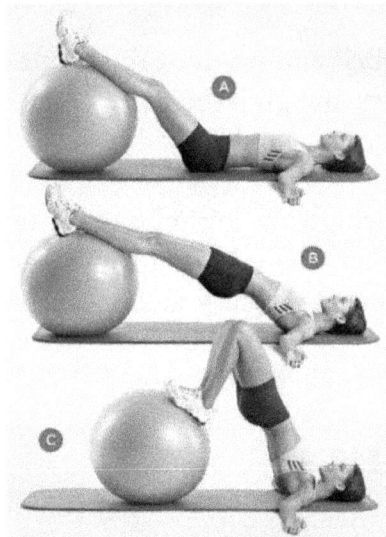

1. Lie face up on the floor and place your lower legs and heels on a Swiss ball. Push your hips up so that your body forms a straight line from your shoulders to your knees.

2. Without pausing, pull your heels toward you and roll the ball as close as possible to your butt. Pause for 1 or 2 seconds, and then reverse the motion, by rolling the ball back until your body is in a straight line. Lower your hips back to the floor. Do 8 reps.

Barbell Dead Lift

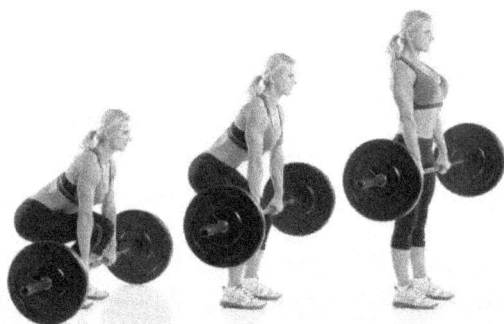

1. Load the barbell and roll it against your shins. Bend at your hips and knees and grab the bar with an overhand grip, your hands just beyond shoulder width.

2. Without allowing your lower back to round, pull your torso back and up, thrust your hips forward, and stand up with the barbell. Squeeze your glutes as you perform the movement. Lower the bar to the floor, keeping it as close to your body as possible. Do 8 reps.

Dumbbell Dead Lift

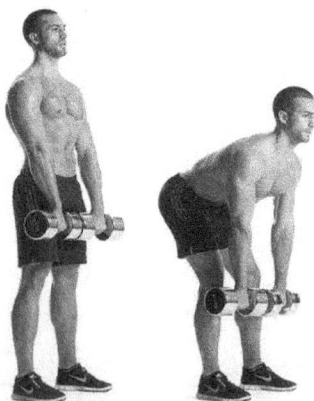

1. Set a pair of dumbbells on the floor in front of you. Bend at your hips and knees, and grab the dumbbells with an overhand grip.

2. Without allowing your lower back to round, stand up with the dumbbells. Lower the dumbbells to the floor. Do 8 reps.

Single Leg Dead Lift

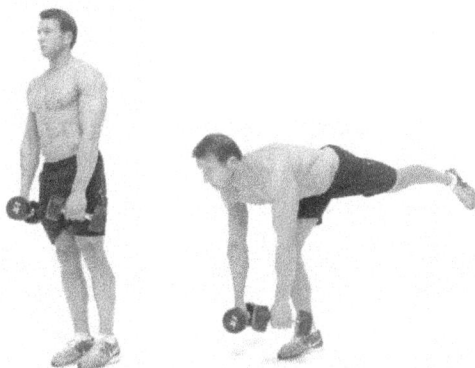

1. Grab a pair of light dumbbells and stand on your left foot. (If dumbbells make this too hard, just use your body weight.) Lift your right foot behind you and bend your knee so your right leg is parallel to the floor.

2. Bend forward at your hips, and slowly lower your body as far as you can, or until your right lower leg almost touches the floor. Pause, and then push your body back to the starting position.

3. If this exercise is too difficult, let the toes of your shoe rest on the floor for balance instead of raising the foot of your non-working leg. Do 8 reps.

Single Arm Dumbbell Swing

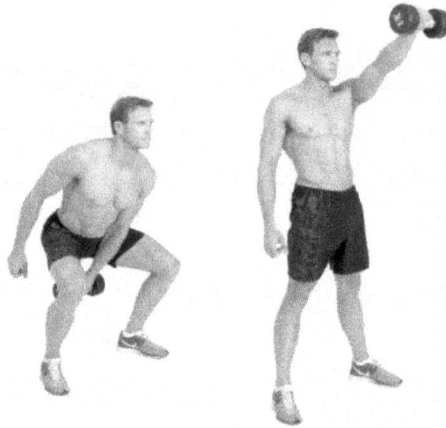

1. Grab a dumbbell with an overhand grip and hold it in front of your waist at arm's length. (You can also do the exercise while holding the dumbbell with both hands.)

2. Bend at your hips and knees and lower your torso until it forms a 45-degree angle to the floor.

3. Swing the dumbbell between your legs. Keeping your arm straight, thrust your hips forward, straighten your knees, and swing the dumbbell up to chest level as you rise to standing position.

4. Now squat back down as you swing the dumbbell between your legs. Swing the weight back and forth forcefully. Do 8 reps.

Clamshell

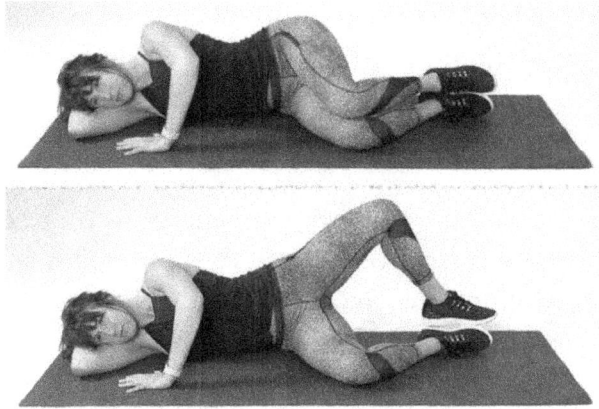

1. Lie on your left side on the floor, with your hips and knees bent 45 degrees. Your right leg should be on top of your left leg, your heels together.

2. Keeping your feet in contact with each other, raise your right knee as high as you can without moving your pelvis. Pause, and then return to the starting position. Don't allow your left leg to move off the floor. Do 8 reps.

Dumbbell Step

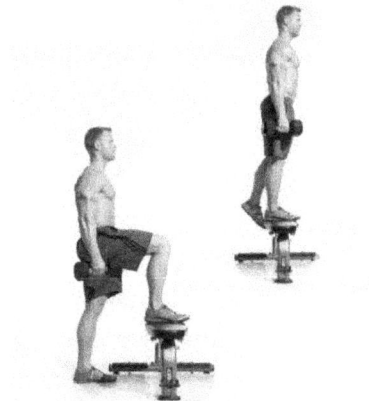

1. Grab a pair of dumbbells and hold them at arm's length at your sides. Stand in front of a bench or step and place your left foot firmly on the step, high enough that your knee is bent 90 degrees.

2. Press your left heel into the step and push your body up until your left leg is straight and you're standing on one leg on the bench, keeping your right foot elevated.

3. Lower back down until your right foot touches the floor. Complete 8 reps with your left leg, and then do the same number with your right leg.

How to Get Jiggle-Free Arms

Many women have problems with their arms; they seem to get flabby really fast. A big problem here is that most women are worried that by incorporating strength training into their workouts they are setting themselves up for big bulging biceps. This is not something you need to worry about – women are not pre-disposed to build bulky muscles and have to work really hard to do so.

When deciding on what exercises to choose, you need to first determine what the problem is – do you have scrawny arms with no definition or is it more a problem with bingo wings? The starter exercise for any arm problem is the pushup. You should aim to do at least five a set. That may not sound like a lot initially but it will be harder than you think. Resistance is key here – it builds muscle strength and tone.

For absolute beginners, start by doing pushups against the wall. Stand an arm's length away from the wall and then lean in. Hold for a few seconds and then push yourself away from the wall again.

The "Real" Pushup

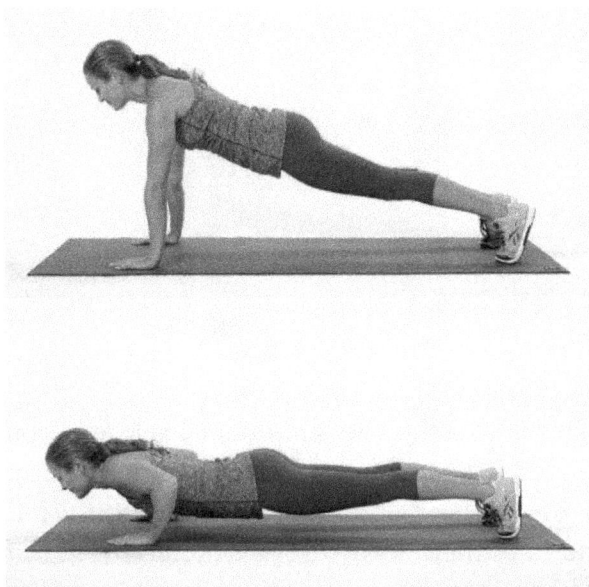

1. Once you can get 5 right, move on to this more advanced version. When you begin this, make sure you get the alignment right by watching yourself in the mirror. It is more important to get the basic movement right than to perform more reps.

2. Keep your hands directly under your shoulders and in line with your chest. Pull in your stomach so your core is steady and ensure that your shoulders and neck are relaxed.

3. In this case, you want to be able to feel the action at the back of the arms to get it right. Keep your body straight and stiff – try to emulate a plank – and parallel to the floor as you push yourself up off the floor. Lower and rest for a few seconds. Repeat 5 – 10 times to start off with and work your way up to 20 reps.

Bicep Curls

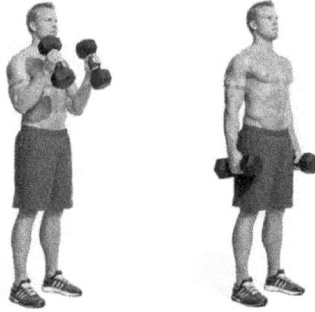

1. The key is to keep the shoulders back and your elbows at your sides. This helps you to really target the arms. Lift both arms together, maintaining this position. Hold for a few seconds and then slowly drop back into the start position.

2. You should be doing about 10-15 reps a set and should work up to 3 sets. The weights used will depend on how strong the muscles are.

3. You want to be just tired enough at the end of the reps that you don't feel that you can do anymore. If you find this exercise too easy, the weights are not heavy enough.

Become Spiderwoman

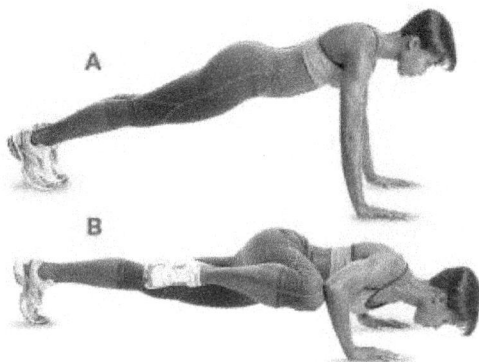

1. These are a little different from your average pushup but can really rev up the results. Start with the advanced pushup but when you have pushed away from the ground, extend your right arm as far as it will go while you bring your left knee in towards your chest.

2. Drop down and do a pushup and then return to starting position before repeating. Repeat on the other side. You should be doing a set of 15 – 20 reps.

Triceps Kick Backs

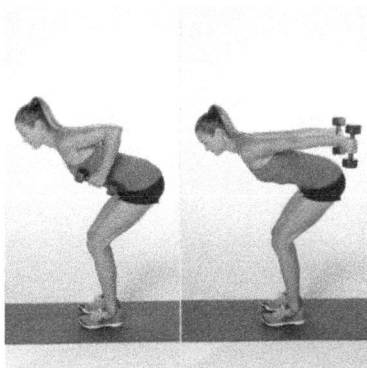

1. If you want to get rid of those bingo wings, this exercise if essential. Stand up straight holding the weight in your left hand. Bend your right knee and lean forward until you are at a 45 degree angle.

2. Again, tuck your elbow in close to the body for support. Extend your arm back as far as you can. You the only section that should move is your forearm. Do 2-3 sets of 15 reps each.

Triceps Dip

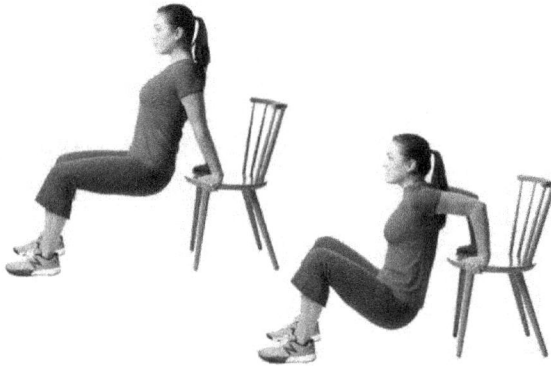

1. This is a bit tougher but works wonders. Sit on the edge of a stable chair. Your arms should be at 90 degrees to the chair.

2. Push yourself off and lower yourself slowly down – make sure that your arms are doing the work – and then push yourself back up again.

Shadow Boxing

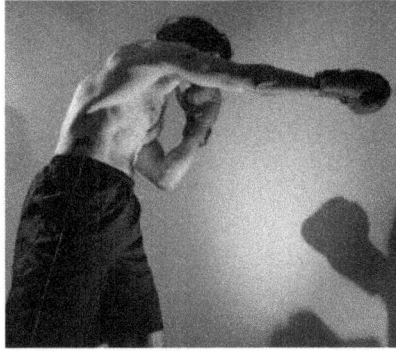

1. Stand with your feet shoulder-width apart and make sure that your knees are loose, not locked into place. Pull in your stomach and then punch across the body. Make sure that the movements are controlled and that your muscles engage. Repeat 15 times on each side, alternating arms.

2. Change position – your arms should be at a 90-degree angle to your body. Punch across the body again. Repeat 15 times on each side, alternating arms.

3. Again, try to take the opportunity to practice some of these exercises throughout the day. If you have a suitable office at work, and a suitable chair, do triceps dips. You can practice your bicep curls when packing away groceries.

Secrets to a Sexy Chest

Working your pectoral muscles is especially important if you want to keep your breasts nice and perky for longer.

For this set of exercises, you want to complete the whole set, without resting in between. Then have a 30 second break before repeating at least 2 or 3 times.

Pushups, Using a Medicine Ball

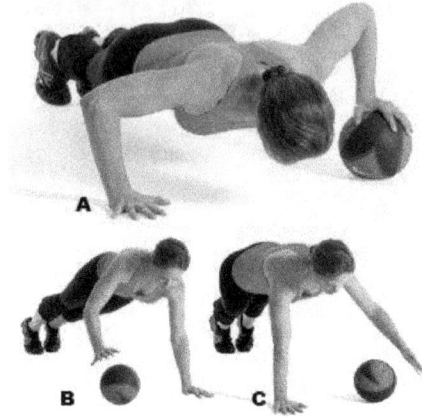

1. Come into a pushup position with left hand on top of a medicine ball, right hand on the floor. Engage legs and stomach in to stabilize core muscles. Keeping the body in a straight line, bend elbows and slowly lower down as far as possible.

2. Press up through both hands to return to starting position. Complete 8 reps on one side and then place the opposite hand on the ball and repeat.

Chest Pass

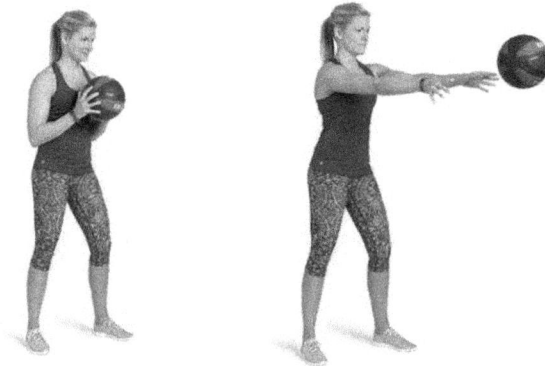

1. Lie face up on the floor with knees bent and feet flat, holding a medicine ball at chest. Keeping lower back pressed into the floor and abs engaged, explosively throw the ball straight up as high as possible.

2. Catch with straight arms and immediately lower back to your chest and repeat. Continue at a quick pace until you have done 20 reps.

Single Arm Chest Press

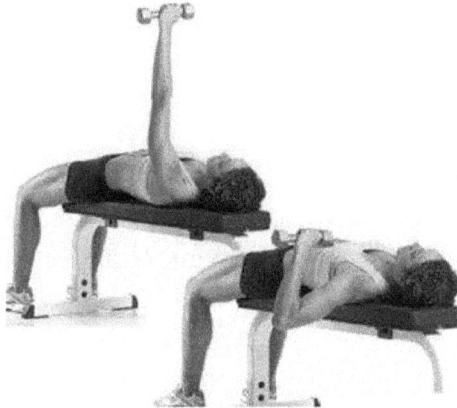

1. You can either do this exercise on a Swiss ball or on a bench. Beginners should start with the bench, as the Swiss ball can be tricky at first.

2. Grab a dumbbell with right hand and lie on back on a Swiss ball. Raise hips so that body forms a straight line from knees to shoulders.

3. Hold the dumbbell at chest and draw shoulder blades down and together. Press the weight straight up and then lower back down to the chest. Nothing but your arm should move.

Complete 8 with right hand and then repeat on the left to complete one set.

Y Raise

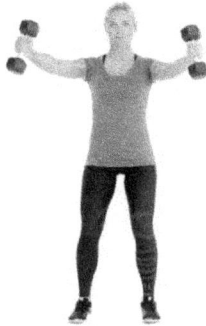

1. Grab a pair of light dumbbells and stand tall with feet hip-width apart, knees slightly bent. Hold the weights in front of thighs.

2. Keeping core braced, draw shoulder blades down and back as you lift the weights above head in a Y position. Return to start at a slow and controlled pace. Repeat 8 times.

Dumbbell Pushup

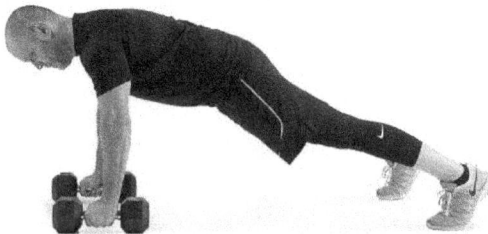

1. Grab a pair of dumbbells and get into straight-arm plank position. Dumbbells should be directly below shoulders, feet slightly wider than hip width.

2. Without moving hips, bend left elbow and lift the weight up to chest, keeping elbow close to body. Slowly lower the weight back to starting position, and repeat on the other side. That's one rep. Repeat 8 times.

Rear Lateral Raise

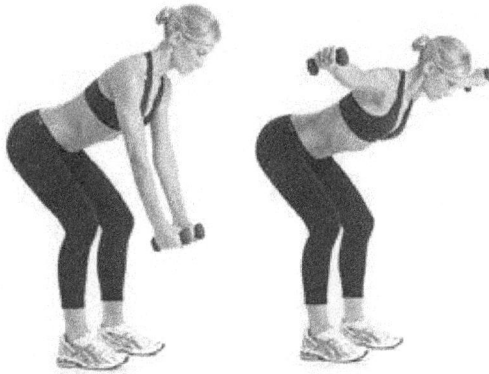

1. Stand with feet-hip width apart, holding dumbbells with palms facing forward. Bend knees, shift hips back, and bring torso close to parallel with the ground.

2. Without moving torso, raise arms straight out to sides to shoulder height. Pause, and then slowly return to starting position. Repeat 8 times.

Wear the Right Bra

This cannot be stressed enough. Nothing damages breast tissue as quickly as not wearing the right bra, especially if you have a large chest.

Without the right support, your breasts start heading south quickly. The bigger the breasts, the more pronounced the problem can be. Most women wear the wrong bra size and use the same bras for too long. Your bras should be replaced every 6 months are so.

It is worth paying a bit more for quality in this instance because the right bra can make a major difference when it comes to what you wear. The bra should lift and separate the breasts. The mid-section should sit firmly in place on the breast-bone and the cups should not gape or bulge over the top.

If you want to look great without a bra on, you need to make to ensure that your bras do support you when you do wear them.

Result Enhancing Rest Days

Your body needs rest as well as workouts. Rest refreshes your mind plus it will renew your enthusiasm. When you exercise, your muscle fibers get tiny tears in them that literally need time to repair. Resting helps to prevent soreness and injury, which will ultimately help you continue on the plan for longer and achieve bikini-beauty success! A rest day certainly doesn't mean lying around in bed or being glued to your laptop.

Here are a few suggestions for your day off:

- Take a leisurely stroll somewhere beautiful
- Do some deep breathing exercises for 20 minutes
- Have a long session in a sauna or steam-room to cleanse yourself of toxins
- Do some very gentle stretching exercises to relieve soreness

- Enjoy an hour in a Jacuzzi
- Have a deep-tissue massage to relieve soreness and shift toxins
- Do some rest-day yoga that will transform your body and spirit.

Read on to the next tip...

Yoga for the Mind & Body

Yoga is an excellent form of relaxation and exercise. It is a type of exercise that dates back over 5000 years and it focuses on strengthening and toning the body, improving flexibility and breathing well in order to boost your physical and mental wellbeing. Regular yoga practice can help to combat high blood pressure, heart disease, joint stiffness, aches and pains, depression and stress. It is essentially a strengthening exercise, which can help you greatly improve your balance, co-ordination and muscle tone, plus it can support weight loss.

Here are 4 simple yoga exercises for a lean body:

Mountain Pose

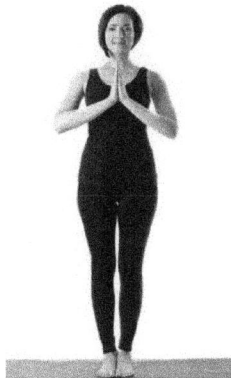

1. Stand tall with feet together, shoulders relaxed, weight evenly distributed through your soles, arms at sides.

2. Take a deep breath and raise your hands overhead, palms facing each other with arms straight. Reach up toward the sky with your fingertips.

Downward Dog

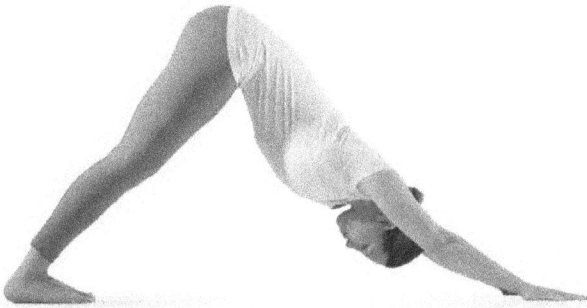

1. Start on all fours with your hands directly under your shoulders, knees under hips. Walk hands a few inches forward and spread fingers wide, pressing your palms into the mat.

2. Curl your toes under and slowly press your hips toward ceiling, bringing your body into an inverted V, pressing your shoulders away from your ears. Your feet should be hip-width apart, knees slightly bent. Hold for 3 full breaths.

Tree Pose

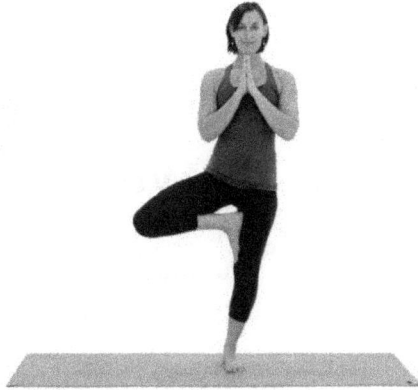

1. Stand with your arms at your sides. Shift weight onto your left leg and place the sole of your right foot inside your left thigh, keeping hips facing forward.

2. Once balanced, bring your hands in front of you in the prayer position, palms together. On an inhalation, extend arms over shoulders, palms separated and facing each another. Stay for 30 seconds. Lower and repeat on the opposite side.

Cobra

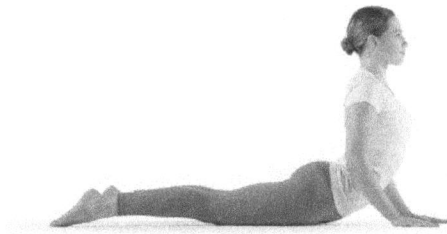

1. Lie face down on the floor with thumbs directly under your shoulders, legs extended with the tops of your feet on the floor. Tighten your pelvic floor, and tuck hips downward as you squeeze your glutes.

2. Press your shoulders down and away from your ears. Push through your thumbs and index fingers as you raise your chest toward the wall in front of you. Relax and repeat.

On-The-Go Workouts

Life is busy. However much you want that perfect body, there is always a lot to do in life, between work, family and friends.

The good news is that you can still fit in a mini-workout!

Here are three routines that anyone can manage on the go – none of them take more than 7 minutes:

Workout A: Quick Interval Training

30 seconds of Jumping Jacks
10 second rest
1 minute of squats
10 second rest
30 seconds of push-ups
10 second rest
1 minute seconds of abdominal crunches
10 second rest
1 minute of step-ups
10 second rest
30 seconds of backward leg lifts
10 second rest
30 seconds running on the spot

END

Workout B: Run, walk, plank

30 second walk

30 second sprint
Repeat 6 times
End with 30 second plank

END

Workout C: Mini Aerobics

30 seconds knee lifts
1 minute waist stretches, reaching up and over, both sides
1 minute running on the spot
10 second rest
30 second plank
10 seconds walking
30 second fast air-punches
30 second squats
10 second rest
1 minute running on the spot
30 second plank
30 second stretching

END

Module 5

Top Tips for Long-Term Body Transformation & Weight Loss Success That You WISH YOU Knew!

The advent of fast-food restaurants and other unhealthy habits have caused many people to put on unwanted fat. The outcries are everywhere that the population of obese people is fast increasing among both the young and old. This has initiated a proactive response from every corner: From the governments, public and private institutions and the experts that an emergent solution be found to stop the problem from expanding. Failure to do so will lead to increase in the number of people suffering from heart-related diseases.

Even though you may not be clinically regarded as obese, you still feel like you are uncomfortable with your current weight and willing to do something about it. That is where this book comes in handy with a complete package of weight-loss procedures you can immediately implement to rid your body of unnecessary fat. The information provided in this book are sophisticated but yet simple for everyone to comprehend. In fact, its step-by-step approach simplifies the process of shedding one's weight without having to go through the hassles of liposuction or plastic surgery.

Here are the undeniable facts revealed in this book:

- That ANYONE can lose weight and change their body in as little as 20 days.
- That a great weight-loss plan should comprise of both dietary requirements and appropriate workouts.
- That the foods we eat are broadly divided into 7 categories, and each category contributes immensely to the metabolic processes happening in human body.
- That a balance diet is needed to burn the fat in human body, and this should be applicable to the breakfasts, lunches and dinners we eat.
- That an appropriate workout/exercise must be carried out to burn those fat in addition to eating a balanced diet: cardio workout and metabolic resistance training are the two most effective workout types, and they simply highlighted in this book.

If you are ready to transform your body, here are **10 tips for success** you may want to have a serious look at:

- First of all, you must have a distinct plan or goal about what you want to achieve as far as shedding some fat from your body is concerned.
- While preparing the meals for breakfasts, lunches and dinners as shown in the book, it is your responsibility to make sure you pay attention to good hygiene. It would be bad for you to contract another disease while preparing any of those dishes.
- In case you are unable to locate the recommended ingredients for the meals in your geographic location, go for something that possesses almost similar properties as the suggested ones. The primary goal is that you can derive some active minerals or nutrients from the ingredients. Most especially if you are allergic to any of the ingredients, seek some medical advice from your physician before consuming them.
- Workouts are good for combusting some fat in your body, but not all of the exercises described here may be OK for you. Maybe you have some disabilities that would prevent you from carrying out some of the exercises. Do not compare the outcomes of your workouts with the others; human bodies are different, and they respond differently to external stimuli.
- Do your workouts in the most comfortable environments for you: use good fitness equipment and make sure you have enough space to move your body around. Do not use any old machines that can inflict some wounds on your body. If you don't know how to use a new equipment, ask for help from the gym trainer or someone you trust understands how the equipment works. One of the mistakes people make is handling the fitness equipment in the wrong way, which will eventually produce nothing but wrong results.
- Drink a lot of water while exercising. You must at least keep the water level in your body in balance. Human body contains about 70 percent of water. Use a clean hand towel to clean your face and body, and make sure you are doing in

a sheltered place as opposed to exercising in the open space. This is to avoid being sun-burnt or gets easily exhausted.

- Make sure you are not indisposed before starting this body transformation program. If you are suffering from any illness, see your physician first and get a clean bill of sound health before proceeding on the weight-loss routine. Failure to do this may force you to abruptly abandon your weight-loss regimens. Some people who failed to heed this advice had found themselves collapsed or fainted during the workouts. So, be safe and take appropriate precautions before things get out of hands.

- Once started, do not attempt to stop for some days before continuing again. It is almost impossible to gauge the efficiency of this plan if you don't execute this weight-loss plan for 20 straight days.

- You need something to motivate you throughout the twenty days: why don't you decide to undertake the weight-loss procedures with someone you are shy of—a friend, colleague, neighbor—who could hold you accountable for your desire to complete the routine. Do not settle for your child or spouse, because they may not be able to compel you to stay on the plan. We all know it is tough doing workouts and preparing meals every day, but once you have a "backer", someone who can push you out of your comfort zone and make you work out so hard, you will be able to transform your body within as little as 20 days.

- Finally, use your discretion in everything you do. There are no guarantees about anything in life. Something that works for someone else may not necessarily work for you. It is your duty to identify which of the meals (breakfasts, lunches, dinners or snacks) is ok for your body and which exercises do not produce painful sensation on your body. Whenever you feel some strange reactions on your skin/body due to the new foods you are eating, contact your doctors for advice about allergy. And if the pain in your body after each exercise persists for up to 48 hours, call up your doctor for an appointment to examine that parts of your body.

You will be surprised how fast you are dropping weight. What separates the facts outlined here from the others out there is that there are no grey areas: every step to be taken is clear, simple and understandable. No expensive clinical procedures are needed, and if any transformation occurs, you will be able to see it with your naked eyes when you start dropping those dress sizes! It is impossible to state exactly how many kilograms you can lose based on this weight-loss plan; this is due to the fact that people have different bodies that respond to things differently.

But here is the rule of thumb: the amount of weight you can lose will surely be commensurable with amount of efforts you put into the workouts and eating balanced diets. Watch your diet during this time, because any mistake of consuming a fatty or high-calorie food may backfire; you may end up making new fat in your body as you struggle to burn the old one. So, consistency is the key here! If you're enjoying this book and would love to let other potential readers know how great it is, please take a few seconds to leave a review on Amazon.com.

How to Look Good NAKED!

We often forget the little things when it comes to how we look, but it is important to take good grooming into consideration. You want to look the best that you possibly can and by implementing a great grooming routine, you can achieve this goal with a lot less effort.

Your Body

If you want truly radiant skin, you have to work at it. Fortunately, if you have already adopted the skin brushing routine previously discussed, you are already part of the way there. Create a great base by:

- Exfoliate your skin at least once or twice a week and particularly if you are going to shave or get a wax. Exfoliation helps to remove dead skin cells that can make skin appear dull and encourages the skin to renew itself. Buildup of dead skin cells on the skin can result in blocked pores and this can lead to acne.

- Use a body lotion every day. Sometimes we neglect this aspect of body care because we feel too busy but it is very important. The best time to apply body lotion is just after you have climbed out of the shower or bath. It helps to lock moisture into the surface of the skin. Rubbing the lotion in does also benefit circulation as well.

- Stretch marks. An unfortunate consequence of gaining and losing weight is that you can develop stretch marks. Using a moisturizing and nutritious Vitamin E oil can help to keep the skin strong and supple and help to reduce the appearance of stretch marks. It is better to deal with these as soon as possible – over time; there is less that you can do to get rid of them. Fortunately, they do fade over time. Having a tan will make them appear less obvious.

- Get a fake tan – these have come a long way since those orange-toned creams that first came onto the market. Tanned skin looks healthier than porcelain white skin and having a tan can help you to look slimmer as well. It is important that you exfoliate the skin beforehand so that you get a nice even tan. You should always practice on a bit of skin that is not visible to see what the results are before applying all over. You need to aim to apply this evenly to avoid streaking. You need to be careful when applying it to areas that are drier – these will absorb more pigment. If it does streak, exfoliate to even it out. You can use a spray tan if you want to in order to make application easier. It is important to stress here that the only safe way to tan is to apply the fake tan. Exposure to the sun will age your skin prematurely and exposure on a tanning bed causes even worse damage.

- There are products on the market now that moisturize the skin and build up color over time. These can be a timesaving alternative to applying a fake tan and will create a more subtle effect.

- Use a bust cream. The skin of the bust is extremely sensitive and needs some TLC. Bust creams help to moisturize but can also help to tone the skin as well. This can help to keep the breasts looking perkier.

- Waxing or shaving. It is not fair that women are expected to keep their legs, etc. shaved and that men can get away with not doing so but that is how life is. Besides, smooth skin is a whole lot sexier. Waxing or using a hair removal cream provides longer lasting results than shaving does, but shaving is quicker and easier. You will have to choose what is right for you. If you are concerned that waxing is going to be painful, time your sessions properly – the week before your period is the worst time to go as your skin is more sensitive. Taking two aspirins before going in can help reduce discomfort during the session. Honestly speaking though, it really is not that bad – it will be over before you know it. Don't apply creams for about a day or so after waxing or shaving.

- Wear a sunscreen when leaving the house and apply to all areas not covered by clothing – the sun is especially damaging to skin. Apply sunscreen more often than you think you should – if you are at the beach, it should be reapplied every time you get out of the water and every half hour or so at least. The level of protection afforded by the sunscreen is based on the application of about two to three tablespoons of the actual product and most of us do not use anything close to that. It is always better to choose a higher

SPF factor. Bear in mind that the SPF factor is an indication of how much longer you can stay in the sun for without burning; it will not provide complete protection. You need to know your own limits when it comes to the sun. The fairer you are, the more sun protection you need to use. Even if you have a darker skin, the sun can cause damage so make sunscreen one of your must-have products.

- You should, however, allow yourself around about 15 minutes of unprotected exposure to the sun once every other day or so. This is necessary to allow the body to produce Vitamin D.

Your Face

Your face requires special attention. The skin on your face is more delicate than the skin on your body and is also more exposed to the elements. A daily cleansing regimen is important to keeping your face looking younger and your skin looking radiant. You should always cleanse your face first thing in the morning – overnight the skin renews itself and, in the morning, you need to clean off the dead skin and any dirt. At night you need to ensure that you remove any traces of makeup and dirt accumulated throughout the day. These can sink into the pores and cause blockages.

Toning the skin is not considered essential anymore. You can choose to tone your skin if you like the feeling of the toner. If it leaves your skin feeling dry and taut, either cut it out completely or change to a milder product. Natural rose water makes an excellent, mild toner. You should follow with a face cream and any specialist products.

The type of face cream that you apply will depend on whether it is morning or evening. It is worth having different products. A night cream will be richer and is best left on overnight. If you are using any products that have retinol in them, you must apply them at night because they can make your skin photosensitive. A day cream is a lot lighter and will normally contain some sort of SPF factor as well. You should also change up your cleansing and moisturizing routine when the seasons change.

In winter, your skin needs more nourishment so a cream cleanser and richer night cream is a good idea. In summer, you want a product that is lighter so that the pores are not blocked. You need to be especially careful when it comes to the eye area. Be careful not to drag at the skin of the eyes as it is very delicate and the first area on your face where wrinkles will show.

When applying eye cream, dab it on with your ring finger – this is the weakest finger and will do the least damage. If you are prone to puffy eyes, try storing your eye cream in the fridge for an instant cooling effect. If the problem persists, you should consider skipping the eye cream in the morning. There are many specialist treatment products out there and some of these can be helpful. My advice is not to go too overboard. A cleanser, a moisturizer, an eye cream and one specialist product should be more than enough. You do not want to overload your skin with too many products.

I have very dry skin and what I have found most helpful is Rosehip oil. I use it at night after I have cleansed my skin. I allow it to soak in for a few minutes, wipe off the excess and then apply my night cream. It's a simple and effective treatment. When it comes to the skin on your face, I favor a simpler approach. It is more important to be consistent than to worry about how much a product costs. Depending on how sensitive your skin is you can exfoliate it every day after cleansing. I use a specialist cleanse that has a mild exfoliating action as well. Once again, if your skin feels irritated or taut because of this action, you should change products.

I also apply a facemask at least once a week. Some beauty magazines advise that you never exfoliate and put a facemask on the same day. I find that the masks work a lot better if the skin is exfoliated first. The key is in choosing the right product for your skin type. Where possible, try and get samples beforehand to test on your skin. By following a good skin care regimen, you are ensuring that your skin looks great naked – even if you are not wearing any makeup at all.

Keeping your face fuzz free is a must – this is easily accomplished and there are many products that you can use at home if you want to. Grooming your eyebrows can also make a huge impact. If your eyebrows are properly shaped, your face will look a lot more open. You should always have your first eyebrow shaping done by a beauty therapist – they will get the basic shape right and from then on it is easy to maintain yourself.

Your Hands

Your hands take a lot of strain. You need to really look after them well. They will often be the first part of your body to show signs of aging – your hands and face are the parts most exposed to the elements. Your face often fairs better because you are wearing makeup and this offers a level of protection.

Ideally speaking, you should be moisturizing your hands every time you wash them. It is a good idea to use a hand cream that has an SPF factor. Your hands and nails are a very important part of personal grooming. Chipped or uneven nails send the message that you are lax in your personal grooming so it is a good idea to keep your nails healthy.

One great product to have on hand, and one that is inexpensive, is glycerin. You can pick it up at the drug store for a couple of dollars and a bottle will last ages. All you need to do is to rub a drop of glycerin into each nail bed every night for a couple of weeks to improve your nails and make them much stronger. It is a bit sticky so let it soak in for a couple of minutes and then wash the residue off.

I had tried all sorts of nail strengthening products but nothing has worked as well for me as plain old glycerin. The other thing that I do every night is to rub a cuticle cream in around the nails. This prevents hangnails from developing – something I used to battle with. Hangnails can be painful and unsightly. I give myself a manicure once a month or so. This also helps to keep the nails looking nicely shaped. A home manicure is simple – start by soaking your fingertips in a little olive oil that you have warmed up.

Rinse it off and then apply a cuticle cream before you gently push back the cuticles. Clear off any residue with an acetone-free nail polish remover and file and buff the nails. Your nails are now ready for nail polish. If you are concerned about upkeep, a clear nail varnish helps to make the nails look finished off without being overdone. You can, alternatively, go to a salon and have your nails done there. If you cannot grow your own nails, gel or acrylic nails are a good alternative. Most important though is to keep the nails looking neat and clean. Your nails should all be the same length and any chipped polish should be touched up or removed as quickly as possible. The plus side of having slightly longer nails? They make your fingers look longer and slimmer as well.

Your Hair

I think a lot of women have a problem when it comes to their hair. If it is straight, we want it curlier. If it is curly, we want it straight. The key to great looking hair is to get the right cut for your hair type. Your hair stylist can advise you on what looks better for your face. Generally speaking, if you have a rounder face, you want to create a bit of length when it comes to the hair. It should be cut either above the jaw line or under it – cutting it on the jaw line can add more width to the face.

The right color can also be very slimming and can help you look more radiant. I am one of those fortunate people who am able to wear just about any hair color. My natural color is a mousy brown so I change it quite often. Color can also help to improve the texture and condition of hair. Proper care is also extremely important when it comes to your hair. You should avoid washing it every day as this can strip out the natural oils. You should always use a shampoo that suits your hair type and you should use a conditioner every time you wash your hair – Even if you have fine hair.

Styling your hair, especially with heated appliances can be very damaging. If you style your hair every day, you can get hair products that help to protect your hair from frying. If you have really thin, fine hair, you can consider having hair extensions put in. Just be sure that you can maintain them afterwards. The better you look after your hair, the better it will behave. A great hairstyle can really lift your spirits and can really help make you look slimmer and better groomed.

Little Extras

If you have a busy lifestyle, you should consider beauty treatments that enhance your natural looks with the minimum amount of maintenance required. Simple tricks like having your eyelashes tinted or having eyelash extensions installed can create a more enhanced look without you having to worry about whether or not you will have time to recreate it every day. These enhancements can be very subtle.

Solving Common Issues That You Have Which MOST People Won't Discuss

This chapter is a quick run-down of some common problems and common solutions.

Cellulite

Nothing can truly get rid of cellulite but you can improve its appearance. Dry body brushing every day can help with this. Before you climb into the shower, brush your body, starting with the feet and working your way up. Use firm brush strokes and brush in the direction of your heart. An easy homemade cellulite treatment can be made using used coffee grounds, olive oil and cling wrap. Mix the coffee grounds from the morning with around about a tablespoon of olive oil and smear onto your thighs. Cover the area with cling wrap and leave for about 10 minutes before rinsing off. Drinking plenty of water and eating more fresh fruit and veggies will go a long way to cleansing your system and clearing out toxins and this will help to smooth the look of the cellulite.

Spots / Blemishes

Whilst we expect to be spot-free when we leave our teens, problem skin can carry on throughout adult-hood as well. You can minimize your chances of developing spots/blemishes by following the right skin-care routine and by providing your body with the nutrients that it needs. You can treat the odd spot by applying toothpaste and leaving it on overnight – this will help to reduce redness and inflammation.

Acne

Acne is a different story - again, it is not confined to teenagers. Acne must be handled properly in order to minimize scarring. Contrary to popular belief, it is not dirt or too much fatty food that causes acne. It is more likely to be a hormone imbalance of some sort. What generally happens is that the skin turns over cells too quickly or that it produces too much sebum or a combination of the two.

A common response to acne is to want to cleanse your face a few times a day to minimize outbreaks. This is more liable to cause future damage and irritate the skin even more. You should wash your face no more than twice a day and should use the gentlest products that you are able to. The best thing to do is to consult a dermatologist and see what they advise. Depending on the severity of the acne, they will advise an appropriate skin care regimen and any medication necessary. You need to nourish the underlying skin and control the acne on the surface and this can be tough.

Flabby Arms

If you want to blast flabby arms, the best course of action is to do pushups. I have dealt with arms in more detail in Chapter 10 but if you want a quick fix, pushups are your best bet.

Muffin Tops

That muffin top that peeks out over your jeans is best dealt with through diet.

Here are some exercises that can prove effective though:

Climbers

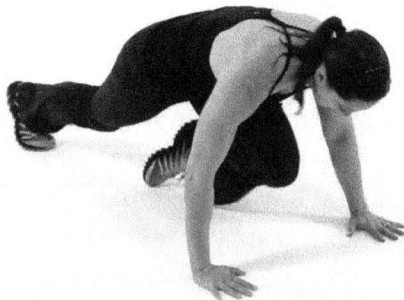

1. Start in plank position, with your shoulders pressed down, and your pelvis tucked.

2. Drive your right knee to your chest, and tuck your chin, keeping your torso and hips stable. Step back to plank and repeat on the other side. Do 15 reps on each side.

Overhead Swing

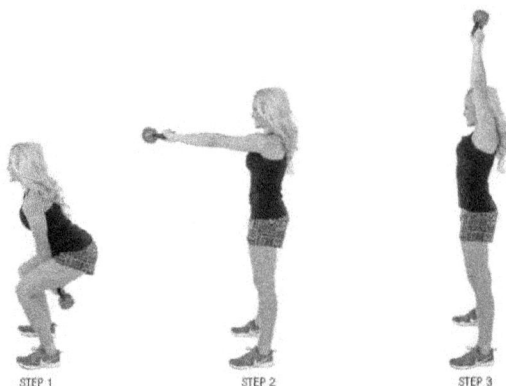

STEP 1   STEP 2   STEP 3

1. Use a kettle bell to blast off those love handles. Put your feet shoulder-width apart with the bell between them, slightly in front of you.

2. Grab the handle with both hands and squat with your hips back. Hike the kettle bell back toward your rear end (don't let it swing all the way behind you; it should stop a little behind your knees).

3. Keeping your back flat and your arms straight, immediately stand up and press your hips forward, swinging the kettle bell upward until it's you're your head. As the bell begins to arc back down, bend your knees and squat, swinging it between your legs. Do 15 reps.

Side-Over Twists

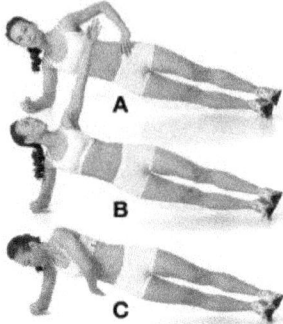

1. Start in a side plank with your left hand on the floor and your right hand reaching to the sky. Inhale and lift your body up until it arcs while reaching your right hand overhead.

2. On the exhale, lift your hips, twist your torso and reach your right arm behind you under your left hip. Complete 10-20 repetitions on each side.

Lateral Bend

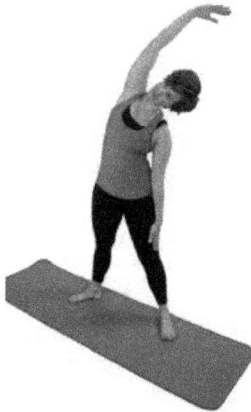

1. This move is a great one to do throughout the day. Stand with your arms stretched overhead. Bend sideways, lift one

knee to the side and pull your elbow to touch your knee. Straighten and repeat on the other side. Do 10 reps on each side.

Love Handles

Love handles can be tough to shift. There really is not much in the way of exercise that can really effectively target them. That said, a good cardio plan will help to boost your metabolism and this will help with weight reduction overall. Cutting back on the number of carbs and junk food that you eat is also essential.

BONUS

The "Wedding Dress" Weight Loss Plan Drop A Dress Size in 7 Days

Is It Really Possible?

Some people would have never come across this amazing weight loss concept before, so you may well be asking yourself – is it even possible to "Drop A Dress Size in 7 Days"? The great news is that, yes, it certainly is! In this section we will show you exactly how to carry out this brilliantly effective short-term plan to transform your body in just 7 days. Not just a little, but a considerable change in such a short time – a whole dress size of difference. This fabulous way to lose weight in just one week is ideal for anyone who wants to look great for an upcoming event.

Perhaps you are planning to go on holiday in a few days and want to maximize your slimming down so that you look spectacular on the beach? You might be about to have a birthday party or go a company ball or another major social event. You could in fact be a week away from attending a wedding – or even be the bride herself! Whatever your reasons and motivations, if you want to lose with in just 7 days, this is the diet for you. You don't have to modify it in weird ways or cross your fingers for luck - if you just follow everything we advise then it WILL definitely work for you, it really is that simple.

What is the Plan?

This 7-day plan is based on eating low-fat, low-calorie, nutrient-rich food. Starchy carbohydrates are kept to a minimum, but not completely cut out, to encourage better weight loss. There are 3 meals a day plus two snacks to enjoy, so you really won't go hungry. We will explain exactly how and why this approach works so well in Chapter 3. Follow the plan just the way we recommend and you will lose enough weight to drop an entire dress size.

What CAN you eat?

You will be amazed at the amount and variety of all the delicious, weight-busting nutrients that can be crammed into only 7 days! You won't miss out on anything that your body needs and you may even be nourishing yourself much better than normal. There is a whole lot of fruit, vegetables and fiber, plus healthy lean meat, so you will certainly not be running on empty. In fact, you are likely to enjoy preparing all the simple yet delectable recipes that we have included in this book. Don't forget, you even get to snack!

Who is this weight loss plan designed for?

This plan is for absolutely anyone who wants to drop a dress size in just 7 days. Or tighten their trouser belt – no reason why guys can't follow the plan too! If you are looking to shed some weight fast but in a healthy way, then you have chosen the perfect plan.

That said, it is not for everyone without reservation. If you have any underlying health problems or are in any doubt about the suitability of the program for your health situation, please consult your doctor before embarking on this or any weight loss program.

Are there any side effects or downsides?

If you follow the plan exactly, there will be no significant negative effects. On the contrary, you are likely to be feeling better than ever during and after the 7-day diet! The only aspect to consider is that this weight loss plan has been especially designed to work quickly and effectively over a short period of time. It is not meant to be followed in the same way for 6 months, for example.

However, it certainly will be possible to adapt the principles to a longer-term mode of eating once the 7 days are up and we will discuss how later in this book. Take time to read and absorb that post-plan advice as it will help ensure that you do not gain back any weight.

What do you have to do?

Each day you simply select one breakfast, one lunch and one dinner from the recipes in the later chapters of this book. You can also enjoy two snacks from the list of ideas outlined in Chapter 9. In addition, you should not drink anything other than unsweetened herbal tea or water. We recommend that you aim to drink at least eight glasses of water per day.

How to Drop a Dress Size!

In this chapter, we take you step by step through the exact way that you can successfully *Drop A Dress Size in 7 Days*.

All you have to do is follow these steps.

10 Easy Steps to Help You Drop a Dress Size in 7 Days

1. **Measure Up** - Take a measurement of your body before you begin. Then keep a record of them and see how you measure up after the 7 days.

   BEFORE:

   BUST_____

   WAIST_____

   HIPS_____

   You may already know your dress size, but it is a well-known fact that some clothes shops go bigger or smaller than the official measurement.

   So, if you want a reliable guide please use the table below as a guide:

US SIZE	BUST		WAIST		HIPS	
	INCHES	CM	INCHES	CM	INCHES	CM
2	31	78.5	23.75	60.5	33.75	86
4	32	81	24.75	63	34.75	88.5
6	34	86	26.75	68	36.75	93.5
8	36	91	28.75	73	38.75	98.5

US SIZE	BUST		WAIST		HIPS	
	INCHES	CM	INCHES	CM	INCHES	CM
10	38	96	30.75	78	40.75	103.5
12	40	101	32.75	83	42.75	108.5
14	43	108.5	35.75	90.5	45.75	116

2. **Think about your motivation** – A spot of mental preparation at this stage can make all the difference to your chances of true success. Think positive, get set, be totally honest and prepare to shine. Write down your own personal answers to these key questions:

Why am I planning to drop a dress size?

What are the possible pitfalls that I must avoid in order to maximize the results?

What is my number one aim through doing this program?

Keep a note of your answers to these questions and refer to them during the 7 days if you feel you are starting to lose motivation. Once you have clarified for yourself why you are going to follow the program, you will find it far easier to motivate yourself.

3. **Next, check-off some of the many benefits of losing weight:**

- Look totally amazing – slimmer, younger, fitter, healthier and more attractive.
- Dramatically cut your risk of cancer, heart disease, stroke, diabetes and other potentially fatal diseases.
- Get a real buzz from fitting into your favorite smaller-size clothes again, or treating yourself to new ones – it is an outstanding ego boost!
- Start positively vibrating with fresh energy and love being able to enjoy more activities.
- Eliminate toxins from your system with a healthy, low-calorie, low-fat, high-water diet.
- Enjoy glowing skin and a stunning, refreshed complexion.
- Benefit from better digestion – if you have had any internal issues they may simply melt away after the next healthy 7 days.

4. **Browse through the recipes** – Chapters 6 through 10 offer a superb selection of recipes for breakfast, lunch, dinner and snacks and each meal is given its own chapter of recipes. Simply pick one breakfast, one lunch, one dinner and two snacks per day. There are enough recipes for all 7 days, although if you particularly like one recipe option, please feel free to repeat your choice and eat it another time as well during the week. You have to eat them at regular intervals throughout the day, giving yourself at least 3-4 hours between each meal.

5. **Once you have had a chance to review the recipes, take a look at the shopping list and mark off all the ingredients you will need to buy.**

    We have not specified strict amounts as that will depend on the choices you make and whether you prefer certain recipes above others. If you intend to try every single recipe during the 7 days, then simply buy everything on the list – it is all there!

6. Next, go shopping.

Fun! All you have to do is buy according to the handy list. However, there is one important additional note to consider when you are shopping. Do aim to buy the best quality fresh ingredients that you can afford. This does not always have to mean that you buy the most expensive food there is, although we recommend organic options whenever possible and this does tend to come with a higher price tag.

It is always worth buying organic fruit, vegetables, cereals and meat if you can possibly afford it. It has been widely debated whether eating organic fruit and vegetables is any different to eating regular produce that has been grown with pesticides and other chemicals. Honestly, it really is different – fact.

Organic fruit and vegetables have been grown in accordance with very strict guidelines to ensure they remain chemical-free. The resulting produce is much higher in antioxidants and much lower in its levels of toxins, metals and pesticides. Not convinced? Check out this study by The Organic Trade Association. They found that the significantly higher levels antioxidants in organic crops included:

- 19% higher levels of phenolic acids
- 69% higher levels of flavanones
- 28% higher levels of stilbenes
- 26% higher levels of flavones

- 50% higher levels of flavonols
- 51% higher levels of anthocyanins

All of these antioxidants have been shown to lower the risk of heart disease, brain diseases and certain cancers. Switch to organic fruit and veg and you will increase the amount of antioxidants you take in by up to 40% - with NO more calories. That's a great reason to go organic when you grab the Shopping List in Chapter 10!

7. **Begin!**

Once you have all your, hopefully, organic food, you need to start the plan. Eat the meals according to the guidelines, i.e. 3-4 hours apart and including the two snacks per day. You can now add a couple more important tips (below and in later chapters) that will turn your week from okay to terrific!

8. **Drink a lot of water** – Few of us drink as much water as we should to stay healthy, and in fact, many people suffer from dehydration in the majority of their working days. They drink little water but do not realize why they feel lethargic, or even sick, and find it hard to lose the excess pounds.

Water feeds our metabolism and flushes out unhealthy toxins that poison our system. We need more water in our lives – or specifically in our bodies – to function well. We are made up of 60% water. We need to keep ourselves constantly topped up with H_2O in order to be able to enjoy the very best of health and lose maximum weight.

So, promise yourself that you will drink at least 8 glasses of water every day during the Drop A Dress Size in 7 Days plan. Not only will it help you to lose weight, but you will also be blown away by how lovely your skin starts to look.

9. **Keep on movin'** – To maximize the effects of this outstanding weight loss plan, it should be twinned with our special exercise plan. This plan involves working out at least 4 times during the week, using slowly controlled toning exercises that work your muscles on a deeper level, build strength, and crucially boost your metabolism to the max.

   We won't outline every exercise that you have to do right here as we go into them in detail in Chapter 4. Trust us though – you will love them and they will make a real difference.

10. **The 7 Days Are Up!** – Once you have completed the steps for this plan, you will notice a significant difference in how you look and feel compared to the start of the week. However, the mirror does not always give the full picture; so make sure you celebrate your transformation by measuring up once more and noting just how much you have lost:

    AFTER:

    BUST_____

    WAIST_____

    HIPS_____

Congratulations!

By this point you will have been through everything you need to do to Drop A Dress Size in 7 Days, so all you have to do to enjoy the results to the max...show yourself off, get into those skinny jeans and spread the word about what you have achieved!

The SECRET of the Plan

Many people are amazed by this plan. They simply can't believe it is possible. After all, shouldn't losing weight be painful and stressful, with weeks of going hungry and many failed attempts to show for every lost pound? The answer is a resounding NO!

Once you learn the secret of this plan, it will all become crystal clear. The plan is not based on chance, luck or superstition. It is solidly founded on reliable biological principles that will ensure that you get the results that you deserve with this superb diet.

So... What's the Secret?

Okay, since you've asked, let's look at why this diet works every time, when followed corrected. There are three pillars to this diet. The low-calorie aspect, the low-fat aspect and the fact that both strategies are supported by calorie-burning, toning exercise. The trick to understanding why these approaches work is not just to understand each one in isolation, it is to recognize that they get brilliant results when working *in combination.*

In addition to these three pillars, the structure of this diet ensures that your metabolism is kept working at its peak, thanks to thermogenesis and to consuming the right amounts of food that support and promotes a faster metabolism. How does the structure do this? Part of the answer lies in the fact that it is essential to eat every 3-4 hours.

In this plan, you never wait too long before the next snack or meal, which has two consequences. First, you are never tempted to gorge on junk due to hunger. Second, you are eating at exactly the perfect intervals to keep those metabolic fires burning.

Why Does It Work?

Unless you are an expert in nutrition, it can be hard to understand precisely why the principles of this plan work every time. So, here is some more information outlining why eating this way works so well for weight loss.

The Low-Calorie Factor

If you understand the calorie principle then you will be several steps nearer to controlling your weight for good. Calories have been discussed in all kinds of ways, but in reality it is very simple. As time passes throughout a day, we eat a lot of food and at the same time we burn calories every day. We must also remember that the drinks we drink can also be very high in calories. Alcohol, for example, contains more calories than carbs.

So, taking into account everything that we consume, food and drink alike, whether we gain or lose weight is all simply a question of balance. If we consume more calories than we burn it will definitely lead to weight gain. If we consume fewer calories than we burn, then we will lose weight. An average man needs around 2500 calories a day to maintain his weight. For an average woman, that number is around 2000 calories a day.

Some plans recommend that you reduce just 600 calories per day. This is shown to result in anywhere from 1-2lbs of weight loss for a slightly overweight individual. Obviously these numbers are all dependent on the individual, what they consume, and how active their lifestyles are. It is not recommended that anyone consume less than 1000 calories per day when trying to lose weight. But the beauty of this plan is that you do not have to constantly count the calories as we have done that for you. Losing weight is well worth the effort and not just for looks. When we carry excess weight we are at far greater risk of a wide range of serious health problems.

First, when we eat and drink more calories than we need, our bodies store the excess as body fat. Fat can be very dangerous for our health, particularly the extra pounds of fat that so many of us can carry around our belly area. If this weight gain goes unchecked and continues over time then we will become overweight, and can even become obese. Being overweight or obese causes an increased risk of type-2 diabetes, heart disease, stroke and some cancers. Many adults in the US need to lose weight, and to do this they need to eat and drink fewer calories. Combining these changes with increased physical activity is the best way to achieve a healthier weight. Remember, achieving a healthy weight is all about striking the right balance between the energy that you put into your body, and the energy that you use.

To lose weight, you have to use more energy than you consume in food and drinks throughout the day. This weight loss book makes this easier for you as it changes your eating habits and encourages physical activity in your daily life. Stick to it strictly for 7 days and you will certainly lose weight. However, there is much more to it than that. Now let's take a look at the type of calories you will be consuming for 7 days.

Low-fat Food

It makes sense to most people that if you don't want to be fat, then you should probably eat less of it, right? This is common sense... but it is not the whole story by any stretch of the imagination. There are different types of fats and they act within your body in very different ways...

Everyone needs some fat as the body requires some fat to function properly. It is a small amount of healthy fat that helps the body to function at optimum levels. But remember the calorie/energy-burning balance. Fat is very calorie-dense - every gram of fat contains 9 calories. What does that mean? Let's compare it to other macro-nutrients:

Protein: 1 gram = 4 calories
Carbohydrates: 1 gram = 4 calories
Alcohol: 1 gram = 7 calories

Eat too much fat and, at 9 calories per gram, it will obviously be fattening. However, not all fats stack up the same nutritionally and some fats are better for you than others.

Unsaturated Fats

These include both monounsaturated and polyunsaturated fats. Polyunsaturated fats come from plants and include olive oil, corn oil, and canola oil, among others. If you are trying to lose weight you should really stick to this category of fat. You will be pleased to note that the majority of our recipes that require fat specify that you use one of these healthier fats.

Saturated Fats

Saturated fats come from animal products, for example meat and dairy foods. They increase the risk of heart disease because they raise the "bad" LDL cholesterol in the body. Only 10% or less of your daily calories should be from saturated fats. The American Heart Association recommends even less — 7 percent. However, this is as part of a normal, daily maintenance diet. If you are trying to actually lose weight then of course it should be far less if possible.

Trans Fats

Quite simply, these are the worst types of fats to eat and too many of them can impact hugely on our health. Trans fats can be found in products like margarines as well as in many unhealthy snacks such as processed foods including cookies, cakes, pies, ready meals and potato chips. Trans fats come in many disguises but they are basically created when liquid oils are transformed into more solid fats, sometimes called "partially hydrogenated oils". This is commonly done to increase the shelf life of packaged food and it is a dangerous feature of processed, packaged, unhealthy foods. Trans fats can actually raise your bad cholesterol and as such, many medical experts recommend that you avoid them altogether.

Why A Low-Fat Diet Works

On a low-fat diet, you restrict your calorie intake through fat to a lower than normal percentage. For example, on a normal weight-loss diet of 1,200 calories, you will limit fats to only 20% of total daily intake. This basically means that you can have 240 calories, or 26 grams, of fat each day, with a maximum of 120 calories, or 13 grams, coming from saturated fat. That leaves you with nearly a full 1,000 calories to "consume" on protein and carbohydrates. However, this plan is no ordinary diet.

For a start, we encourage the consumption of some low-fat dairy products. They are rich in calcium and vitamin D and these help preserve and build muscle mass. The higher the percentage of fat in your body and the less muscle, the worse your ability to burn calories. Conversely, having a good muscle mass is essential for maintaining a super-efficient metabolism. We also recommend that, in order for this superb weight-loss program to work at its best in a short space of time – you eat less than the standard amount of even the healthy fats. This way you will be burning stores of unwanted fat to make up the difference, which you will be hugely grateful for when you see how great you look after just a few days!

Not to Forget... The Thermogenic Factor!

Certain foods have a very high thermogenic effect, so you literally torch away the calories as you eat. Other foods contain nutrients and

260

compounds that add kindling to your metabolic fire. Feed your metabolism with these wonderful dietary additions.

- **Whole grains**: When your body tries to break down whole foods your body burns twice as many calories. This is especially true when it comes to those foods that are rich in fiber, like oatmeal and brown rice. If you only consume processed foods, you lose this advantage, as well as lots of fiber and vital nutrients.

- **Lean meats**: Lean protein really is the dieters' friend and it has a very high thermogenic effect. Did you know that you burn about 30% of the calories the food contains during digestion? This means that a 300-calorie chicken breast requires about 90 calories to break it down. Eat lean and burn, baby, burn!

- **Lentils:** One cup of lentils packs in an amazing 35% of your daily iron needs. This is fabulous news, since up to 20% of us are iron- deficient. When you lack a nutrient, your metabolism slows down because the body's not getting everything that it needs to work efficiently and to lose weight, your body needs to be working as efficiently as possible.

- **Hot peppers:** Want to add some real fire to your metabolism and burn calories as efficiently as possible? Capsaicin, the compound that gives chili peppers their heat, warms up your body, so that you burn off additional calories. You can get it by eating raw, cooked, dried, or powdered peppers. Some of our brilliant recipes include a little chili, or if not, you can up your burn rate simply by nibbling a tiny raw chili pepper alongside your chosen food.

- **Green tea:** It is a proven fact that green tea can help you dramatically lose weight, more than any other drink (apart from water). Drinking four cups of green tea a day, helped people shed more than six pounds in eight weeks, as it was reported following a study in the American Journal of Clinical Nutrition. There is a compound in the green tea called EGCG and it temporarily speeds metabolism after sipping it. To up your intake, keep a jug of iced tea in the fridge.

- **Fabulous Fish:** Salmon is high in protein, and a fatty fish such as salmon contains essential omega-3 fatty acids. These have been shown to regulate a vital body hormone called leptin, which is involved in the regulation of energy. When leptin is efficiently regulated and present in the body in lower levels, this hormone an associated with an increased caloric burn. Tuna is also an excellent source of omega-3s and should freely be enjoyed as part of a healthy diet.

The Carbs Question

On the weight loss plan, we include reduced levels of wheat intake. This means less white bread and pasta - for several reasons. First, starchy carbohydrate acts just like sugar in the body, spiking the blood and causing a surge of insulin... The result? The body is commanded to hold onto the calories as fat. Not good!

In this diet, the starchy carbs, things including but not limited to bread, noodles and pasta, potatoes, root vegetables like parsnips, and rice, are strictly limited. This is with good reason as they are not only calorie-dense, but they will simply cause you to feel bloated and are converted straight into fat if you eat too them in great quantities (and aren't able to burn the resulting energy).

On the flip side, if you cut them out completely, then you can find that you simply put weight straight back on when you start eating them again. We want your weight loss to be both highly effective and lasting, so we encourage you to enjoy light amounts of carbs as part of this diet. You will find that this helps to curb your hunger and also keeps your metabolism burning.

Staying Off the Caffeine

Throughout the 7-day period, you also need to avoid all alcohol and caffeine. Alcohol is bad for dieting all round, as it is very high in calories at 7 calories per gram, plus is drains your energy, acts as a depressant and hampers your metabolism. Additionally, you will be exercising regularly and this is terrible for your health if you try to do it under the influence of alcohol (or have any traces of alcohol in your blood)!

Also, during the 7-day diet do not drink regular coffee or tea at all as these are packed with caffeine, which we all know is a stimulant. Despite being great in some instances, for the goal we have for these 7 days it won't be that great of a help. However, herbal infusions and rooibos/red bush tea are absolutely fine. Naturally, you should also make sure that you avoid all energy drinks as they are simply packed with added sugar, often labeled under other names like 'glucose' and so on.

You Will NOT Starve

By this stage you should have taken a look at all the recipes in this book. We hope the variety and great tastes on offer have come as a pleasant surprise! After all, the meals in this plan are not designed to starve you skinny. The length of this diet may be short, but the results are meant to be more than short-term.

Starving will only backfire because you will be hungry and miserable all the time and more likely to eat unhealthy snacks or overdo the portion sizes. You should note that when you starve-eat-starve-eat your body goes into total crisis mode and it immediately stores fat.

It is a survival response – we were not meant to starve. Our poor bodies do not know we are aiming to look thinner and does its best to hold onto every single calorie, so the cruel result is that you pack on a load of extra weight, so you starve again and the cycle goes on and on...

This slimming plan is completely different. It is low in fat and low in calories, so the weight comes of quickly, very quickly, but it does not starve you to an unhealthy degree, so your body thrives rather that fights to survive. You will not starve on this diet. Remember, you will be eating two snacks a day in addition to three full meals per day and your body really does not need more than that if you follow our recipes. On the contrary, this weight loss plan will not give you too much or too little of anything – you will receive just enough to *drop a dress size in 7 days*, period. Consuming all those empty calories in sugary, fatty or processed foods will not trip you up.

However, you will certainly not starve either - you will receive all the best nutrients and plenty of fiber and water. Your digestion will function properly, you will burn plenty of calories and your metabolic rate, boosted by the exercise you are doing, will even increase. Stick to the program for 7 days and the pounds will fall off.

The Water Secret

You are advised to drink a lot of water throughout the 7-day slimming program. And it will work wonders for your weight loss, skin, digestion and general health. If you drink little and often, you will find it easier. Try starting your day with a refreshing, rehydrating, detoxifying, cleansing, enjoyable glass of water and lemon. Keep a bottle of water with you wherever you go. Drink some peppermint tea after your evening meal (it is wonderful for digestion) and try to end the day with more water, perhaps in the form of another soothing herbal tea like chamomile. Water has an amazing amount of benefits for the body.

First, it keeps you completely hydrated, which is absolutely vital for your body to function properly. Water also flushes out the vast majority of toxins and it does it healthily and effectively. Plus, it keeps your metabolism all fired up and your digestion working at its peak, two benefits that are the best possible news for anyone who is trying to lose weight.

There is even more good news when it comes to drinking plenty of water. Water fills you up brilliantly so that you are far less tempted to cheat with fatty or calorific snacks. It also fully quenches your thirst, whereas alcohol, coffee and sodas, even diet sodas, just pretend to, while dehydrating you even more - and best of all water contains zero calories. Have a love affair with water throughout the whole of the next 7 days and afterwards as well. Try to drink 6-8 large glasses each day.

Speed Up Your Transformation

Now that you are getting closer to beginning your transformation of a whole dress size – it is time to consider that other pillar of weight loss success. That's right, the exercise factor. Almost anyone who has lost weight, however much and however quickly, has explained that it has, in some respect, been down to eating less and moving more.

This slimming plan is no different in that regard. In fact, it focuses on exercise even more carefully than usual as you only have a week to play with. So, what is the most effective form of exercise to change your body shape and burn ample calories in just 7 days? Is it doing 20 crunches, going for a walk, or jogging? No, no and no – they are all great forms of exercise, but for this program we need exercises that will create a long, deep calorie-burn and work your muscles effectively.

Plus, the whole workout has to be more compact because life is busy and there may not be time to exercise for one or two hours every day. A current workout that has proven very popular and effective relies on carrying out different exercises intensively but for just 90 seconds. That's right, just a minute and a half of work, but each exercise is so well-targeted that it can make a whole of difference to your body

How Does the 90-Second Workout Work?

The fun thing about the 90-Second Workout is that instead of doing 30 press-ups or 40 crunches over and over, you do each exercise just once, or once on each side. Unbelievable!

To make it work, you spread the movements over 90 seconds, even though it is just one rep, so that the muscles work really hard to tighten and tone your physique. So – one long rep instead of 20 or 30. Sounds totally doable, right? Well it is – and it is also fun and very effective indeed. Follow this routine for the first 3 days of the plan. Then, have Day 4 off, then do the routine again on Day 5, Day 6 and Day 7.

Safety First

A few notes before you start exercising. While this routine is designed to help you, it is important not to stress your body to the extent that you do yourself an injury. If you are not currently fit, or if you currently have an injury of any kind, please consult your doctor. If in doubt it would be better to delay following the plan until you are given permission to continue by a medical professional.

The Exercises

There are just four main postures to carry out in this routine, although some exercises are comprised of a couple of parts. They will work your body deeply, burn calories and build muscular
266

strength... which means you will burn even more calories. Muscle tissue burns more calories than fat, even when you are resting. According to scientists, 10 pounds of fat burns 20 calories when you are resting, while 10 pounds of muscle in a person of the same size burns 50 calories. Exercise is quite simply the gift that keeps on giving!

Exercise 1 – The Super-Squat

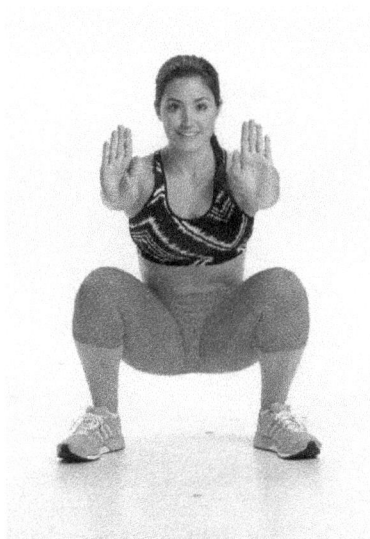

This exercise works the legs and butt to perfection.

1. To achieve the initial position, stand with your feet shoulder-width apart and your arms raised to shoulder height, balancing carefully. Slowly bend your knees and lower your body, being careful to keep your hips over your heels and your back straight.

2. When you have reached one-third of the way down, pause and hold your position for a full 10 seconds. Carry on descending 2 inches, lower 2 inches, raising your heels if you need to. Hold this position for a further 10 seconds. Repeat

this lowering and holding technique three more times, each time keeping position for a full 10 seconds.

Note: Make sure you hold your belly in and keep your shoulders back as you perform this exercise. It will make a lot of difference.

Exercise 2 – Backwards Fly with Ball

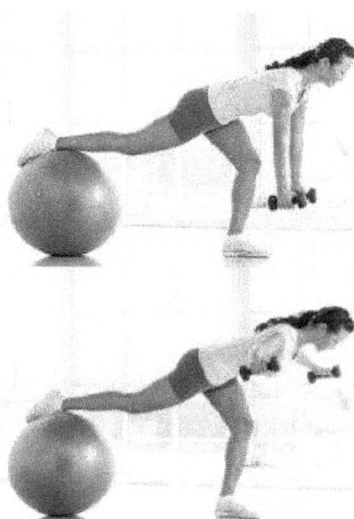

This exercise may seem difficult at first but don't give up. It is really worth mastering this move as it thoroughly works the thighs, butt, back, arms and shoulders.

There are two parts to this exercise. You will need two dumbbells weighing 5 to 8 pounds and a medium to large sized exercise ball.

1. Begin with one dumbbell in each hand and your right leg lifted behind you so that the top of your right foot rests on the exercise ball behind you. Bend your left knee to 45 degrees, rolling the exercise ball backward and hinging forward until your back is parallel to the floor and your arms are hanging straight down.

2. With your elbows slightly bent, raise each arm a few inches and hold the position for 10 seconds. Then raise your arms 2 inches more, and hold for another 10 seconds. Repeat this pattern of lifting and holding 3 more times, until you end with your arms at shoulder height.

    Then slowly lower your arms a few inches, hold for 10-seconds and do this 3 more times. Now repeat the whole exercise standing on the other leg.

Note: It will help you a great deal if you draw your abs in and up and keep your hips square. Don't worry if you wobble, just regain your balance and keep going.

Exercise 3 - Ab-Fab Rotations

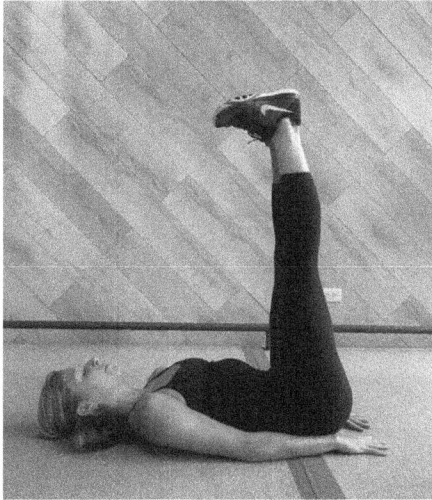

This exercise is performed lying down, but don't be fooled into think this is some kind of rest!

1. Lie down on your back with your legs lifted straight up. Your arms should reach out to either side with your palms down.

2. Lower both your legs a few inches to the left, then hold that pose for a full 10 seconds. Lower your left 2 inches more to the left, and then hold for another 10 seconds. Repeat the lowering and holding 3 more times, until you end up you're your legs hovering just above the floor.

   Raise your legs back to the center in 4 increments, raising and then holding for 10 seconds each time. Now repeat the whole exercise on the opposite side.

Note: Make sure you keep your abs drawn in as you move, to protect your lower back and also keep your right shoulder down to prevent strain.

If you want to mix things up a bit, you can also try rotating your legs left and holding them just a few inches from the floor for a full 45 seconds. Then return to the top position and repeat the hold on the right side.

Exercise 4 - Fly the Bridge Backwards

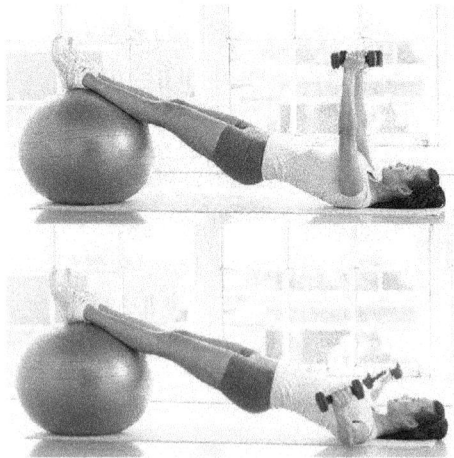

This outstanding exercise is not always easy at first but persevere as it is worth getting right. It works the hips, hamstrings, butt, chest, arms, and shoulders, so it is a pretty comprehensive exercise all-round. You will need the dumbbells and the exercise ball once again.

1. Lie flat on your back with your feet on top of the exercise ball and your legs straight, being careful not to lock your knees. Hold a dumbbell in each hand, with your arms raised over your chest. Press your heels into the ball, and slowly lift your hips so that your body forms a straight line. Do try and keep it as straight as possible as your hips may be tempted to sag – don't let them!

2. Bend your elbows slightly, then open your arms a few inches to the side; hold this position for a full 10 seconds. Open your arms 2 inches more, and hold again for 10 seconds. Repeat this opening and holding 3 more times. Then close your arms in 4 increments, each time with holding period that lasts 10 seconds.

Note: This is not the easiest, but it is worth it. Don't worry if you need to take a quick break partway through. Just stop, breathe deeply and get going again as soon as you are able.

Time Out

That's it, you're done. This set of exercises will really reach the parts that other workouts can't reach, so expect to feel like you have worked hard. However, it has only taken a few minutes to achieve some serious muscle flexing and calorie burning. Now just unwind and look forward to repeat the routine every day, apart from Day 4 of the plan.

Top Tips to Drop a Dress Size FAST

So – you know what food you are about to start eating and why. You know the right exercises to perform and how. You have a water bottle on standby. You are feeling positive, motivated and excited. But here's the thing – there are only 7 days to drop the weight, so what other things can you do to turbo-charge your weight loss and achieve maximum results? Read on, you might be surprised...

1. **Try to minimize your sugar and carb intake as much as possible.**

   They may be the first 'treats' we all reach for when we are stressed, upset or tired and as they tend to be highly processed and packaged we don't usually even have to go to the trouble of cooking them ourselves. Sugary snacks and too many carbs really are your enemies for the duration of this diet. You may feel you need them, but you don't – they may give you a sugar rush, but you will feel horrible when you crash back down to earth. If only for 7 days, just don't do it, it's not worth it. That is not to say you can never ever eat a donut again, of course you can. But after dropping a dress size and looking better than ever you may not even want to anytime soon.

2. **Make sweat your friend**

   That's right, time to really sweat. We have looked at the exercises and if you do those right then you should certainly get pretty worked out, but you can sweat even more than that! Time to rediscover the pleasures of a great session in a sauna, or even to try it for the first time. You may already know that our skin is our largest organ and largely responsible, along with our liver and kidneys, for the elimination of toxins. We need to appreciate our ability to sweat and make the most of it. After all, sweat contains measurable amounts of toxins that have been safely removed from the tissues.

When you sweat, you are detoxifying your body and when you do that, it encourages weight loss. We know that sweating is good for us. When it doesn't occur in a situation that we find socially embarrassing, we can even relax and feel the impurities being drawn out of us, a wonderful feeling of being cleansed. Sweating helps clear out nasty toxins and excess fluid and can be a great starting point for a healthier lymphatic system and a faster metabolism. So, why don't we spending more time sweating our troubles away? Well, not everyone has a sauna at home, or even in their nearest gym. But during this 7-day program, it would be great if you could have at least two sauna sessions.

Some people also find the high temperatures uncomfortable. However, they should be aware that there are now many more low temperature saunas. A typical sauna is anywhere from 160 – 180°F, but the less common "thermal chambers" are set to around 100 – 120°F, so you can realistically stay in there for much longer than the usual 15 minutes or so and therefore you will sweat more. More sweat means more depuration, or washing away of toxins. The toxins essentially get carried away by the water that our body produces, like rivers washing dirt and litter away. Sweat works in the same way.

So, do enjoy the pleasures of a good sauna. If you can, try to line one up after you do your exercise routine, as you will sweat even more. Alternatively, go straight from the office and relax in the heat – the important thing is just to sweat! Saunas can play a really important part of any diet or detox regime. They will only boost your progress and make you feel good. Just make sure you remember to shower thoroughly afterwards, before you simply reabsorb the unwanted toxins.

3. Detox to the max

A key reason why your body is holding excess fluid and extra fat is due to a build-up of harmful toxins. Modern life is pretty toxic, so it can be pretty hard to avoid coming into contact with substances that poison our system – skin creams, cosmetics, alcohol, medicines and drugs, detergents, perfumes... we are bombarded with toxins every day, even before we take a mouthful of food that contains, pesticides, additives, preservatives and other dubious, potentially carcinogenic substances.

If you smoke as well, it is at least ten times as damaging... Wouldn't it be great to stem the endless flow of toxins, even for just one week? Well you can, as much as possible – view this 7-day plan as an opportunity. Drink the recommended amounts of water (starting the day with water and lemon), do the exercises and follow the diet closely as discussed – this will all help detoxify your system. But on top of that you can add in not only saunas but also something called dry skin brushing to physically move the toxins out of your system.

4. **Dry body brushing**

The benefits of dry skin brushing include increasing the circulation to the skin and therefore reducing the appearance of cellulite. Skin looks smoother, brighter and clearer. Dry skin brushing may also help rid the body of annoying ingrown hairs. However, the main point of this activity is to detoxify the body. Dry skin brushing helps to hugely improve blood circulation and lymphatic drainage. It releases toxins and promotes the discharge of metabolic waste. Also, dry skin can clog the pores and therefore brushing dead skin cells away helps your skin to absorb nutrients in a far more efficient manner.

All this means that after a little dry brushing the body can function more effectively. In turn, this means that you can lose weight much more quickly! Enjoy a better detoxification and simply get into a routine of dry brushing every morning before your shower or bath. It is very straightforward, does not take much time and you don't need membership of some exclusive spa. All you need to do is buy a natural bristle brush with a long handle so you will be able to reach all areas of the body.

Here's exactly how you do it:

- Take your brush and work it around your body in gentle circular, upward motions, followed by longer, smoother strokes.
- When you perform a dry body brush, always start at your ankles and work upwards in slow firm movements towards the heart. There is a logical reason for this - the lymphatic fluid (which critically fights infection and disease) flows through the body towards the heart. It is therefore very important that you move the brush in the same direction.
- There is one exception to this rule, which applies to your back. Brush in firm strokes from the neck down to the lower back.
- From your ankles, slowly move up to your calves and then brush your knee area, thighs, stomach, back and arms. Do not brush too hard over the softer and more sensitive areas of skin located around the chest and breasts. Also, make sure that you never brush over inflamed or broken skin, sunburn, or skin cancer.
- When you have given your body a thoroughly good brushing always jump straight into the nearest shower in order to wash away all those dead skin cells and harmful released toxins. Remember, leave toxins on your skin for too long and they will simply be reabsorbed into your system.

- Top tip: If you would like to stimulate the skin even more and invigorate your blood circulation, then play around with the temperature of the shower. Turn the control from hot to cold and cold to hot a few times, which will not only give your pores a work out that tingles, it will also make you feel really alive!
- After you have showered, do apply a wonderful, rich and nourishing moisturizer to your damp skin. Do keep it unfragranced and as natural as possible if you can, otherwise what was the point of all that detoxing? For best results use pure cocoa butter, or coconut oil, while argan oil is outstanding for problem areas like scars or stretch marks.
- Repeat the dry brushing routine as often as you like. If you keep it up for each of the 7 days and then carry on afterwards you will transform the quality of your skin as well as your body,]

5. De-stress

Question: Is the rumor that stress makes you fat actually true?
Answer: It certainly is!

Why exactly does stress make you fat? It is something that feels as if it is true and we have all had those days when we have been over-burdened or strung out and eaten exactly the wrong thing because it was hot, quick and greasy. That is one way that stress makes us fat – we are unhappy and so we eat to soothe our emotions rather than to fuel us with nutrients. Or more accurately we overeat to soothe our emotions...

Plus, when we grab that burger, it is not just high-calorie and high-fat, it is also high in sodium. Sodium, or salt, causes you to retain water and it is found in large quantities in highly processed or fast foods. However, there is even more to it than that. Stress itself can also cause you to hold onto fluid, making you feel constantly puffy and bloated, not a great feeling at all.

Finally, stress leads to the production of hormones that slower your metabolism and reduce the speed of weight loss. So how can you get rid of stress? In several ways:

- ***Consider meditation.*** This ancient form of deep relaxation can be very therapeutic and is highly recommended for people who are feeling stressed or who suffer from what can be described as 'a chatty mind'.

- ***Write a journal at the end of every day.*** Unburdening your main of the day's events can feel very rewarding and reassuring. Do it long-hand with a pen rather than online in order to relax properly as the light emitted from computer screens and other devices can cause insomnia. Conversely, writing in the old-fashioned way is relaxing and sharing your troubles, secrets and thoughts with a confidential book is very soothing indeed.

- ***Face the problem.*** If you have a specific issue that is making you stressed, face it head-on before attempting a weight loss program. Share your troubles with a partner, co-worker or friend, or even simply write a list of the issues with ideas about how to tackle it. It the problem is a real biggie that can't be addressed in a week, you can still take positive steps. Contact someone who can help – a doctor, lawyer or therapist. Get an appointment in the diary and a load will be lifted from your shoulders.

6. Ditch the salt habit

We have touched upon this when looking at stress – too much sodium in the diet can lead directly to water retention, which means a puffy, bloated body. Not good. What is good is the fact that you hold the solution in your hands, literally. Put down the salt for a week. It will not add calories, but it will add to the amount of water that you ultimately retain, so who needs it? You can still season your food and you will be surprised how much flavors can be enhanced by other herbs like parsley and coriander, or spices like cumin, or the brightest flavor hit of all - a little squeeze of lime and a couple of thin slices of chili – delicious!

7. Care for the inner you

No one ever succeeded in a weight loss plan without a clear idea in their own mind about why they are doing it in the first place. We have touched upon this in the earlier preparation stages but it really is worth re-emphasizing. Get your head straight. Dig deep, give yourself a little tough love... whatever it takes. Keep a note on you at all times that reads:

"I am doing this because _____"

It could be something simple like "because I have a wedding to go to next Saturday" or it could be something much deeper. It doesn't matter, it's not a writing competition. It's all about you, so make it honest and make it personal to you. Pay attention to your state of mind during the 7 days. If you feel you are getting down, take steps to pep yourself up, with a beauty treat, going to see a movie, or just having a good chat with a friend. If you are in great shape in your head you can get into great shape in terms of your body.

8. Favor only the good fats

Healthy omega-3 fats can help you lose weight. Linseed, walnuts, mackerel and sardines among other foods all help produce the fat-burning enzyme PPAR-alpha. This enzyme is known to help prevent the storage of fat on the body. Be very sure to understand this – eating a little good, natural fat will not result in piling on the pounds. However, in this low-calorie, low-fat diet, even the good fats are to be consumed in moderation.

9. Start the plan on a Thursday

Sounds strange perhaps, but research proves that you're twice as likely to stick to a diet when you get nearer to the weekend. The pressure is off but the motivation is on, so boost your willpower and forget the tyranny of Manic Mondays for good!

10 . Laugh it up!

Just when you thought we were getting too serious... This is a little reminder that getting slim and gorgeous really is fun! The diet plan is fantastic and that, along with the exercise, will help you drop a dress size, but you can make certain lifestyle changes that may help. Laughing properly, with deep 'belly laughs' - are exactly that; they work and strengthen your abdominal muscles. Think about it – that has to be the most fun workout ever!

Still, life isn't always a barrel of laughs, so you can't be expected to be constantly rolling around in a state of mirth. But you can stay upbeat, be more open to laughter and encourage the release of those stress-busting endorphins that come with a good chuckle. There seems to be a pattern forming here when it comes to getting the right state of mind for weight loss and it appears to be 'don't worry, be happy'!

11. Focus on your food

Don't be confused – this does not mean worrying about more creative food ideas – we have all that covered for you in later chapters. But it does mean that you should concentrate on what you're eating, when you are eating it. Don't eat in front of the TV, don't eat on the run and definitely don't shovel food into your mouth at the cinema without thinking... It's time to be mindful about what you eat.

Sit and eat at the table, the old-fashioned way. It has lots of advantages, not least making you realize in both body and mind that you are eating. Dress up the table if you like. Put away your smartphone. Chew properly and take your time. It will be worth it – studies show that people who eat while texting or watching TV may overindulge by up to 30%. Chances are they are so engrossed in the movie that they don't even realize what they are doing! So – focus on your food. You will eat far less and enjoy it much, much more.

12. Get green power

There are certain health supplements that you can take which may help you lose weight. Seek these ultra-healthy supplements out at your nearest health-food shop to boost you 7-day plan. They tend to work by either speeding up your metabolism or cleansing your body of even more toxins:

Green coffee – This contains a caffeine-based ingredient that speeds up fat metabolism so you lose weight quicker.

Spirulina – This is a type of micro-algae that can be used to maximize the detox effects of the Drop A Dress Size in 7 Days plan. It is a super-effective and healing detoxifying agent which taste like harmless vegetable matter and comes in powder form.

Chlorella - Natural superfood chlorella has exceptional detoxifying properties that help to eliminate mercury and other toxins. It also comes in powdered form, you can mix it with the spirulina powder and add water, the drink it down for a pre-breakfast detox boost.

Green tea – Don't forget to keep drinking this to give a boost to your metabolism.

Flax seeds – Not technically green, but still plant-based so they count. Flaxseeds contain many highly beneficial nutrients, including vitamins, minerals, omega-3 fatty acids and fiber, which normalize the work of the intestine.

Flax absorbs the toxic compounds from the food, cleans the intestines and supplies the body with lecithin, which stimulates the metabolism of fat. Not bad for a few little seeds!

Sprinkle them raw over some of the delicious dishes in the recipe section for added crunch, taste and most importantly a whole lot more nutritional and detox power.

13. Don't hate your scales.

You may be measuring in inches and your dress size, but if you are determined to lose weight, you will need to start thinking of your scale as a friend, not an enemy. Weigh yourself once a day, first thing in the morning after going to the bathroom and getting undressed. This way your numbers will not be swayed by water weight and clothing – every pound counts. A week is a short time, but if you track your results and stay motivated you may be amazed how the pounds can come off quickly.

14. Embrace the power of positive thinking and post little notes with your goals written on them in spots you'll see, especially on the fridge. Other good places include the top of your computer screen and the bathroom mirror – wherever you will spend some time looking each day. Write what you want to do and why, for example:

"I want to drop a dress size in 7 days so I look great at my best friend's wedding."

Make it short, clear and honest. Research conducted by the Dominican University of California showed that people who wrote down their goals, shared them with a friend, and then followed up with weekly updates were, on average, 33% more successful than those who didn't write down their goals or share them with others. You may only have a week but stay motivated every day and beyond by writing down your goals.

15. Don't be tempted to skip

If you are going to succeed on this 7-day plan, you have to trust it. Stick to it just as it is written and you will lose weight. You may think that it would be quicker and more effective to take a shortcut, in other words, by skipping the odd breakfast or lunch.

Our advice? Don't do it. You may end up taking in fewer calories that say, but you will also have slowed your metabolism back down and, if you go for too many hours without eating, you may even have kicked your body into starvation mode. You really do not want to do that, as it is in this mode that the body hold onto every single calorie for dear life and stores as much fat as possible, just in case the body won't receive any food for a while. So – don't skip breakfast, lunch, or dinner and eat both your snacks. Your appetite will be sated, you won't cheat on the diet and your metabolism will not slow down, jeopardizing your diet.

14. Get app happy

You don't need to do this to succeed in this diet plan, but if you are a lover of tech and are glued to your smartphone anyway, you may find it motivating and fun...

Track your calories with a great app such as My Fitness Pal. You can even scan barcodes that will tell you the precise amount of calories, although as you are eating fresh that will hopefully be on a packet of carrots rather than a bag of pretzels. Calorie-counting may lose its novelty after 7 days, but if you love your stats and want to see reports that show how much energy more energy you are burning than consuming, try an app like this one.

15. Ban the booze, period

This is one that many dieters dread, but it is very important. Do not be tempted to have a glass of wine, or a beer, under any circumstances during the 7-day plan. Alcohol is simply too calorific, plus it is a toxin and it will stop you from exercising properly. In addition to that it may weaken your willpower and encourage cravings for high-salt, high-fat foods...Bad news for dieters all round. Give your liver a break and just ditch the booze, totally and willingly, for the whole week.

Some people who worry about this tip more than any other report back afterwards and have no idea what they were worried about. You really can go liquor-free for a few days. Then, when you are feeling fresh and great, you will simply wonder why you didn't do it sooner!

16. Look for ways to fidget.
Researchers discovered that people who tap their feet, fidget, and move around more burn 350 extra calories a day—that's more than a major fast-food joint's cheeseburger! If you do not fidget naturally, just keep one getting up and moving around throughout the day, stretch, jump, bounce and dance around your home, to increase your calorie burn rate throughout the day.

17. Move around the office more.

You may be stuck at a desk for the vast majority of the day, but you can still make calorie-burning differences with a few small changes to your behavior:

Ditch emails on Friday: Change the habits of a working lifetime and walk over to your colleagues instead as once used to happen in every office, when everyone was slimmer! If you are in a big office this is all the more reason to do it, you might really clock up some miles.

Use a standing desk: A modern solution to the problem that millions of us who are stuck at a desk all day face. Essentially, this higher-level desk is designed to be used while standing, which keeps you more active, toned and burning more calories as well.

Alternatively...

Sit down but use a Desk Stepper: This is a clever machine that is becoming increasing popular and is quite widely available. It simply goes under your desk while you remain seated. It works like a stair stepper and you tread on it while you do your normal day's work. The beauty of this is that it is not as conspicuous as a standing desk, but will still work off a decent number of calories – over 90 in 20 minutes. Well worth investing in this little piece of kit when you add up how much you could lose over a week.

Have active meetings: If your schedule includes lots of sitting through meetings every day, change it up. If just two of you are having an internal chat, well why not agree that you will stroll as you talk. You can cover some ground and it might even keep you more switched on and inspired for longer as the blood gets moving around.

Make it a fitness-friendly office: Don't sit among a bank of computer screen with everything at arms' length like most of us do. Try shaking things up a bit so that you simply have to move to carry out your job. Of course, you may be busy, but fit, active people get more done in the long run, so it is worth the extra effort. One small example would be to move your trash right away from you so you have to walk back and forth to your desk.

Better still, get rid of it altogether so that you have to go to another part of the building entirely. You may be astounded at how much office carpet you cover with this move. It does pay dividends.

Have many water cooler moments: Don't sit with a huge bottle of mineral water at your desk. No we are not suggesting that you keeping topping up with gallons of coffee instead! Keep a small glass handy and keep getting up to refill it at the water cooler which is hopefully a bit of a walk away. This might sound like a waste of time, but it is in fact a clever way of building in the regular breaks from your desks that doctors and health professionals agree are much better for your continued health.

Plus it has other benefits too – you will keep yourself hydrated with nice, cool, fresh water and you are highly unlikely to miss out on any of the best office gossip for which the water cooler has deservedly become so famous!

Get a Park Buddy: At lunchtime, don't be tempted to hide behind your screen eating a sandwich and sitting still for the fourth hour in a row. Why not ask a friend if they would like to get some fresh air with you in the local park? It might just be that you go for a casual stroll or a brisk walk, or you might play some sports there even simply jumping after a Frisbee (great exercise) – whatever makes you happy and gets you moving.

Breakfast Recipes

The phrase 'A Breakfast of Champions' is worth remembering as the fittest and most active people tend to swear by eating a good morning meal to set them up for the day. Breakfast revs up our internal engines and fires up our metabolism so that we burn calories more quickly for the rest of the day – provided we eat the right food. It is vital to choose the best options first thing in the morning. After all we are literally breaking our fast after a night of sleep and our bodies are crying out for the right fuel and hydration.

The first thing you should consume upon waking is a large glass of still, warm or room temperature water with a slice of lemon in it. That will hydrate and refresh you beautifully, as well as helping to cleanse and detoxify your system. Next comes breakfast. But what do you eat when you want to Drop A Dress Size in 7 Days? We have made it super-simple for you. Just pick one of the 7 breakfast recipes in this chapter and prepare it just as we instruct. Then you will receive the perfectly balance of calories and nutrients in low-fat form. The recipes are so quick, easy and delicious, you will probably keep on making these breakfasts after the 7 days are up! We have consciously only given you the 7 best recipes that we could devise, so that life remains far simpler and you don't have to browse through page after page, building a super-long shopping list. Just choose one recipe per day and if you come across one that you are not keen on, just repeat one of the other recipes. The official Shopping List in Chapter 10 states all the ingredients that you will need.

Whatever you do, don't ever be tempted to skip your nutritious breakfast. A number of respected studies prove the link between obesity and people skipping breakfast. Conversely, people who are trying to lose weight are more likely to succeed when they eat a good, healthy breakfast. You can't get healthier than these low-calorie, low-fat meals, which also punch well above their weight in terms of taste.

Enjoying a good breakfast will not only fuel your metabolism, it will give you the energy to exercise properly. The workout you will be performing on most days will be most effective when you are well hydrated and nourished – and breakfast eaters exercise more effectively. Also, when you eat a decent breakfast you are less likely to 'cheat' on your diet as you won't feel hungry.

While starving ourselves can sometimes seem like a short cut, it rarely is because the body responds in the end by clinging on to its fat stores, making it much harder to lose the unwanted weight... There is never any need to skip a meal during the diet, so simply relax, browse the recipes and enjoy your great breakfast. It will ultimately help you to look and feel fantastic!

Very Berry Muesli

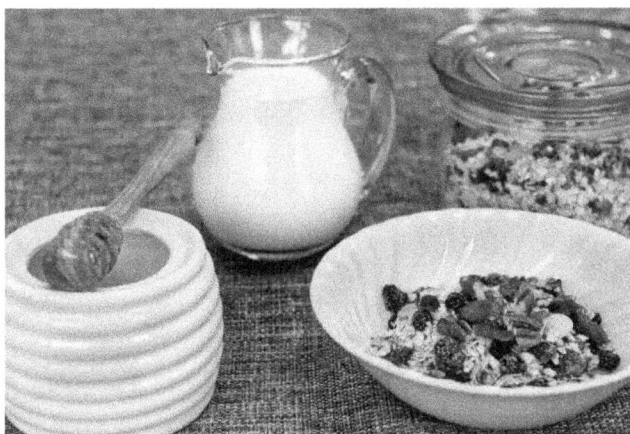

Muesli can make a great breakfast, particularly when it is the coarse, unsweetened kind, which goes heavy on the wholegrain and heart-healthy oats. It provides slow-burning fuel and will keep you feeling satisfied until lunchtime for relatively few calories.

Meanwhile, the fat-free natural yoghurt delivers outstanding health benefits. The calcium boost will support excellent bone health, which is great news at any age. Also, a respected study showed that dieters who ate some yogurt daily lost more belly fat, and retained more lean muscle than those in the same study who did not eat yogurt, so eat up.

Finally, the raspberries are a superb fruit addition, providing plenty of vitamins and nutrients... but there is even better news for slimmers. Scientists have found that phytonutrients in raspberries can help to boost the rate at which fat is metabolized – have you seen all the raspberry ketone supplements that have taken the dieting industry by storm? Have some - fresh, low-calorie and delicious. Wash it down with a glass of orange juice to send your vitamin C levels sky-high.

Ingredients

- 1 oz. unsweetened muesli
- 1 tbsp. fat-free natural yogurt
- A handful of raspberries
- PLUS 1 glass unsweetened orange juice, ideally freshly squeezed

Method

1. Choose your favorite bowl and pour in the muesli – remember, do not add sugar or honey. Top the muesli with the tablespoon of yogurt and the raspberries. Enjoy your fruity bowl along with your glass of orange juice.

Tomato Toast

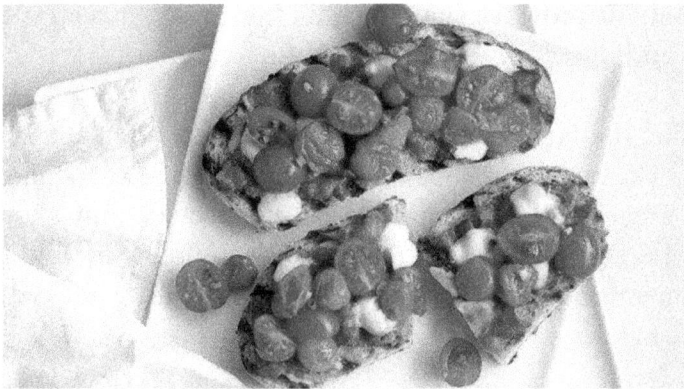

This quick and easy breakfast recipe is super-tasty and as healthy as anything, so enjoy it without guilt! Bread can be controversial among dieters, but as long as it is a good quality whole-meal variety, it will be perfect for this 7-day plan. We firmly believe in the nutritious power of high-fiber whole grains, but they do contain starch to do make sure you stick to just one slice, not three!

Tomatoes are an everyday superfood. They are so good for us, but we sometimes take them for granted. Ripe tomatoes deliver a wonderful flavor and are bursting with lycopene. Lycopene has be found to help prevent certain cancers, as well as diabetes and heart disease. It can also boost male fertility, support your eyesight, prevent skin aging and protect it from sun damage, plus it helps to prevent osteoporosis. This unfussy recipe shows tomatoes off to their tasty best.

For the glass of juice, try freshly squeezing your own OJ, or if you have a juicer, try fresh pineapple.

Ingredients

- 1 slice of whole meal bread
- 3 cherry tomatoes
- Freshly ground black pepper (optional)
- PLUS 1 glass unsweetened fruit juice.

Method

1. Lightly toast the whole meal bread in the toaster on the lowest setting. Meanwhile, slice the cherry tomatoes and pre-heat the grill to a medium heat.

2. Take the toast and arrange the cherry tomato slices on top. Place under the grill for 5 minutes, or until the tomatoes have softened and the toast has browned. Remove and eat hot, with a grinding of black pepper, if you wish.

Poacher's Breakfast

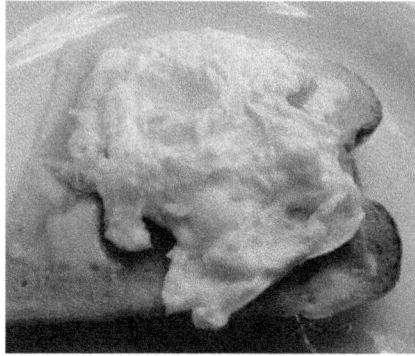

Eggs are a natural, delicious, superfood. Low-calorie and ultra-versatile, they are also protein-packed and highly nutritious – every serious dieter should stock up on plenty of the organic, free-range variety. Nutrients include Vitamins A, B2, B5, B12, B6, D, E and K, plus folate, selenium, calcium and zinc – just fabulous!

Ingredients

- 2 small free-range eggs
- 1 slice of whole meal bread
- 1 drop of vinegar
- 1 pinch of salt (for the water only)

Method

1. First, get the eggs poaching. Put on a medium-sized saucepan of water to boil and add a pinch of salt to it. Make sure your egg is really fresh and crack one into a ramekin or cup. Add a small drop of vinegar to your egg.

2. When the water is boiling, take a hand-held balloon whisk and stir the water to create a gentle whirlpool in the water, which will help the egg white wrap around the yolk.

3. Slowly tip the egg into the water, white first. Turn the heat right down to the minimum setting. Leave to cook for three minutes. Meanwhile, after about a minute and a half has passed, pop your whole meal bread in the toaster, so it should be ready at about the same time as your egg.

4. After three minutes, remove the egg with a slotted spoon, snipping off any straggly edges using the edge of the spoon.

5. Rest the egg to drain onto kitchen paper for a few seconds – this is an important step as a waterlogged dish is unpleasant. Place the egg onto the whole meal toast – no butter – and enjoy it hot.

Tropicana Smoothie

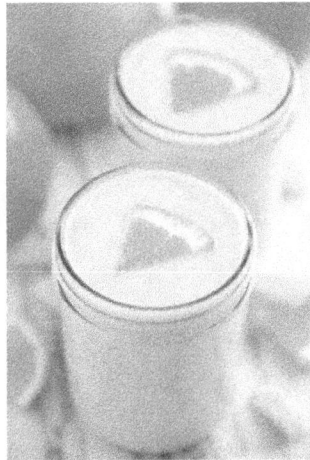

Sometimes you need a fruity start to the day... try this delicious smoothie, which will give you a fantastic dose of vitamin C from the orange, potassium from the banana and plenty of calcium too along with a host of other nutrients. Plus, this tropical concoction tastes out of this world – a real sweet treat that makes a brilliant breakfast on any day.

Ingredients

- 1 large orange
- 1 banana
- 1/4pt semi-skimmed milk
- 1 small pot of natural yogurt
- 1tsp clear honey

Method

1. Peel the orange to remove all skin and pith and peel the banana, then chop them into pieces. Place the fruit in a blender and pour in the milk and yogurt. Whizz it all up in your blender and serve.

New York Summer

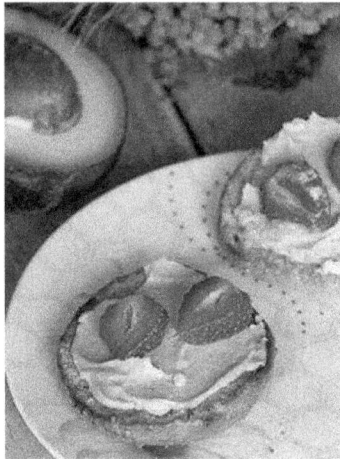

This delicious breakfast is fresh-tasting with the light, creamy cheese and juicy strawberries. The whole-wheat butter-free bagel will provide you with plenty of fiber. Meanwhile, the delectable cream cheese packs a great calcium punch without the usual calories.

Finally, the strawberries are a total superfood – they are packed with antioxidant vitamin C, which boosts immunity, supports your eyesight, helps to combat cancer, stimulates collagen production and much more. Plus, they are very low in calories and high in fiber.

So, as you can see, while this breakfast treat looks and feels somewhat naughty and decadent, it is extremely good for you, so don't hold back!

Ingredients

- 1 whole-wheat bagel
- 1tsp reduced-fat cream cheese
- A large handful of strawberries

Method

1. Slice the bagel into two halves and toast them. When it is ready, spread the reduced fat cream cheese onto the hot bagel halves. Eat hot, nibbling the strawberries alongside as a sweet treat.

Egg and Hummus Breakfast Wrap

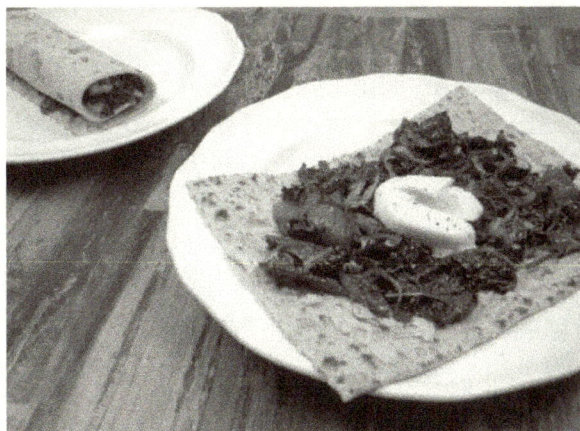

Time for a really wholesome and filling breakfast recipe. This is no ordinary wrap – it is bursting with the protein-packed goodness of eggs and chickpeas, plus nutrient-rich mushrooms and onions for a real hit of savory flavor and tasty textures. The spinach is also a star of this dish – it is a powerful source of both iron and Vitamin C and it cleanses the blood – a great detoxifying leaf.

Ingredients

- 1 whole grain tortilla
- 1-2 tbsp. hummus
- 1 large egg
- 1/4 cup egg whites
- 1/8 cup chopped onion
- 2 button mushrooms, sliced
- 2 cups baby spinach
- 1 tbsp. crumbled reduced-fat feta
- 1 tbsp. chopped sun-dried tomatoes
- Low-calorie cooking spray
- Freshly ground pepper, to taste (optional)
- Hot sauce (optional)

Method

1. Spray the skillet with the low-calorie cooking spray and sauté the onion and mushrooms for 3-4 minutes or until tender and fragrant. Add spinach and sauté the vegetables for a few minutes longer, until spinach has wilted.

2. Add egg and egg whites to pan with veggies and cook for about 2 minutes or until eggs are cooked through. Add a grind of black pepper if you wish. Warm up the tortilla in the oven for a few minutes.

3. Spread a layer of hummus on the tortilla when ready. Place the eggs in the center of the tortilla and top with the sun-dried tomatoes and low-fat feta. Season with more pepper as well as hot sauce if it takes your fancy. Wrap the tortilla up and serve!

Veggie Breakfast Bake

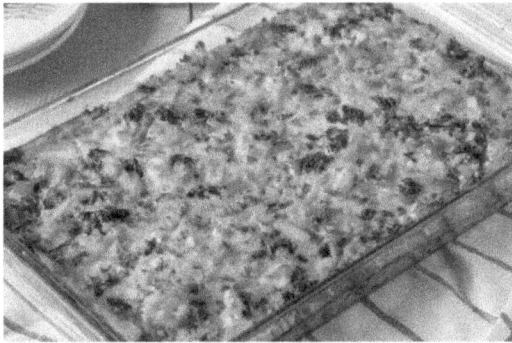

This is the last breakfast of the week, if you select them in order, so it could well take the place of a Sunday fry-up. It is a totally delicious take on a cooked breakfast, with none of the fatty, processed bacon to ladle on the calories. It features the 'everyday superfood' tomatoes, plus powerfully iron-rich spinach and a lovely, large mushroom too. Mushrooms have very few calories and have the added benefit of having been shown in studies to enhance weight loss.

Ingredients

- 1 large egg
- 1 large field mushroom
- 2 tomatoes, halved
- A large handful of spinach
- 1/2 garlic clove, thinly sliced
- 1 tsp. olive oil

Method

1. Heat oven to 200C/180C fan/gas 6. Put the mushroom, tomatoes and slices of garlic into an ovenproof dish. Drizzle over the oil and grind over pepper, then bake for 10mins.

2. Meanwhile, put the spinach into a colander, then pour over a kettle of boiling water to wilt it. Squeeze out any excess water, then add the spinach to the dish.

3. Make a little gap between the vegetables and crack an egg into each dish. Return to the oven and cook for a further 8-10mins or until the egg is cooked to your liking.

Lunch Recipes

Welcome to your lovely lunch section – your choice of deliciously healthy mid-day meals. The recipes include a wide range of flavors and textures so there is no danger of getting bored – it's not all lettuce 24/7. The selection of dished is varied but simple. There is certainly something here that you will enjoy and we hope that you love all 7 dishes on offer. The lunches will give you plenty of slow-burning and healthy energy, plus a kaleidoscope of colorful, flavorful nutrients all for remarkably few calories – the perfect recipe for success when you are aiming to lose weight.

In this chapter, the recipes offer plenty of healthy fiber, in a variety of forms, plus some tasty lean protein. All of the recipes opt for the healthier forms of carbohydrate, so you will be well fueled, but also nourished to just the right degree. You won't feel hungry and stressed-out on this diet – just stick to the plan and enjoy some great food as you Drop A Dress Size in 7 Days. It is essential that you enjoy a good lunch every day. Regular good food will keep your energy levels up, which is vital for when you are exercising most days. Plus, it will keep your metabolism revved up and burning faster, which is very important for when you want to keep the pounds dropping off.

Finally, it will help to keep your spirits high throughout the week, which will only make your diet more effective. If you are the kind of person who grabs a quick bite on the go at lunchtime and sometimes falls into bad habit by choosing a greasy snack over something light, bright-tasting, properly nourishing and uplifting, then you are in for a real treat. Also, of course you may not want to cook a full-on lunch every day, especially if you are working. So these recipes are simple and light, without skimping on flavor or interest. The majority of them can be made in advance and stored for whenever you need them, or taken to work in a lunchbox, or heated up at the office. When you are devoting your week to shedding the excess weight, then you don't need added complications, just delicious, easy to prepare meals.

Also, do remember that since these lunch recipes are mostly quite high in fiber, you may feel that you are eating more food than usual. This is not the case in weight loss terms – fiber is your friend. It fills you up and helps to look after the digestive system. In fact, you will simply be enjoying, healthy, balanced meals with just a fraction of the calories. So, get stuck in – every recipe here tastes wonderful!

Tricolore Salad

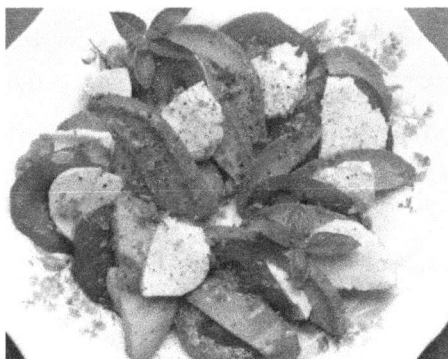

This "three-color" Italian salad may make you do a double-take at first, because it may appear to stray from the low-fat ethos. The great news is that while it has some fat, these are the best types of fat for your health and they may even help you to lose weight. Fresh-tasting, creamy avocados are a real nutritionists' favorite, being full of healthy fats. Twinned with lycopene-rich tomatoes and calcium-packed mozzarella, it helps to make a truly delicious salad, with some crunchy wholegrain crackers on the side.

Ingredients

- 1 small avocado
- 1 tomato
- 2 oz. reduced-fat mozzarella
- 2 wholegrain crackers

For the oil-free dressing

- 1 tbsp. balsamic vinegar
- 1 tsp. wholegrain mustard

Method

1. Slice up the tomato, avocado and reduced-fat mozzarella. Mix the balsamic with the mustard, beating with a fork to thoroughly blend. Drizzle the oil-free dressing, over the salad. Serve your Tricolore Salad and enjoy it with the two wholegrain crackers.

Your Choice Veggie Soup

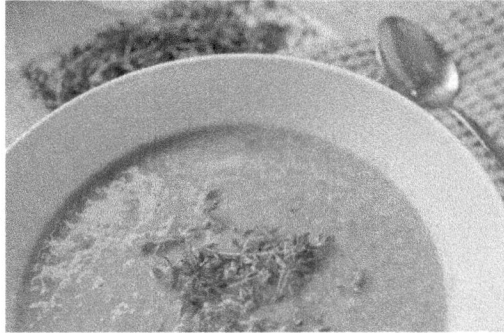

This lunch is great for when you want something warming and wholesome. We call it "your choice" because it is one recipe where, if you fancy, you can take an easy shortcut. If you are pressed for time, or are working during the day, you may want to simply buy a soup. If this is the case, go for a ready-made soup that is high in green veg like kale, not too heavy on the potato and is ideally free from additives and preservatives. If in doubt and if you have enough time, the better option would be to make your down delicious vegetable soup from scratch. Just follow the simply recipe below.

Ingredients

- 7oz zucchini, roughly sliced
- 2oz broccoli
- 4oz kale, chopped
- 500ml stock, made by mixing 1 tbsp. bouillon powder and boiling water in a jug
- 2 garlic cloves, sliced
- A thumb-sized piece ginger, sliced
- ½ tsp. ground coriander
- Thumb-sized piece fresh turmeric root, peeled and grated, or ½ tsp. ground turmeric
- A pinch of kosher salt
- 1 lime, zested and juiced
- A bunch of parsley, roughly chopped, reserving some to serve

- 1 tbsp. sunflower oil
- Plus, a whole-meal roll, to serve

Method

1. Put the oil in a deep pan, add the garlic, ginger, coriander, turmeric and salt, fry on a medium heat for 2 mins, then add 3 tbsp. water to give a bit more moisture to the spices.

2. Add the zucchini, making sure you mix well to coat the slices in all the spices, and continue cooking for 3 mins. Add 400ml stock and leave to simmer for 3 mins. Add the broccoli, kale and lime juice with the rest of the stock. Leave to cook again for another 3-4 mins until all the vegetables are soft.

3. Take off the heat and add the chopped parsley. Pour everything into a blender and blend on high speed until it is a lovely smooth green with speckles of kale. Garnish with lime zest and the reserved parsley, then serve, with a whole-meal roll on the side.

Garden Open Sandwich

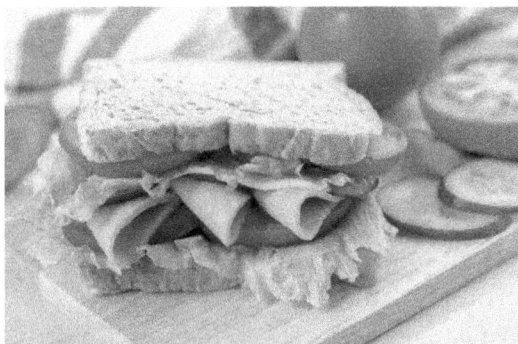

Sometimes you just want fast food. So, go for it! But happily, on this plan, that does not have to mean a fatty burger, quite the opposite.

When you want it fast and flavorsome, try this easy-to-make open sandwich which gives you everything you need in one delicious hit – lean protein in the ham, fiber and many other nutrients in the arugula and tomatoes, plus some wonderful whole-grain bread.

Sticking to one slice of whole-meal instead of two greatly lowers the calorie toll and creates a lighter, fresher dish. You can even eat a calcium-rich, low-fat yogurt straight afterwards if you wish. Just make it quick, easy and totally enjoyable – the perfect workday lunch.

Ingredients

- 1 slice of whole-meal bread
- 2 slices of lean ham
- A handful of arugula leaves
- 2 tomatoes, sliced
- Plus 1 fat-free fruit yogurt for afterwards

Method

1. Lay the whole-meal bread on a plate. Top it with the ham, in ridges if possible for added texture.

2. Scatter over the arugula then top with the tomato slices. It's ready! Don't forget, you can enjoy a fat-free fruit yogurt afterwards if you fancy something sweet but light.

Piri-Piri Prawn Pita

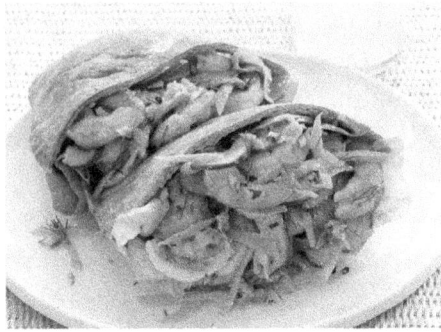

This is a super flavorsome pita lunch. Prawn are delicious, especially when perked up with a spike of chili. Chili pepper is fantastic for speeding up the metabolism, so don't hold back. It's the perfect partner to ingredients on the Drop A Dress in 7 Days diet.

Ingredients

- A large handful of peeled raw king prawns
- 1 small whole-wheat pita bread
- A few leaves of gem lettuce
- ½ red pepper, sliced
- 1 tbsp. fat-free sour cream
- Juice of ½ a lemon
- A handful of mint, finely chopped
- 1 tsp. olive oil
- 1 garlic clove, crushed
- ¼ bird's-eye chili, finely chopped (remove the seeds unless you want it very hot
- Sprinkling of paprika

Method

1. Heat oven to 160C/140C fan/gas 3. Mix the fat-free soured cream with a squeeze of lemon juice, the fresh mint and seasoning, cover and put in the fridge. Put the oil in a skillet

302

and heat it on medium-high. Add in the slices of red pepper and cook them until they start to soften.

2. Meanwhile, wrap the pita pocket in foil and heat it in the oven. Add in the prawns to the skillet, another squeeze of lemon juice, the garlic, chili, paprika and seasoning. Cook and stir until the prawns are cooked through.

3. Remove the heated pita and slice a slit into it. Place it on a plate. Stuff the pita pocket with lettuce, plus the pepper and prawn mixture. Top with the cold, seasoned fat-free soured cream and enjoy.

Cheesy Jacket

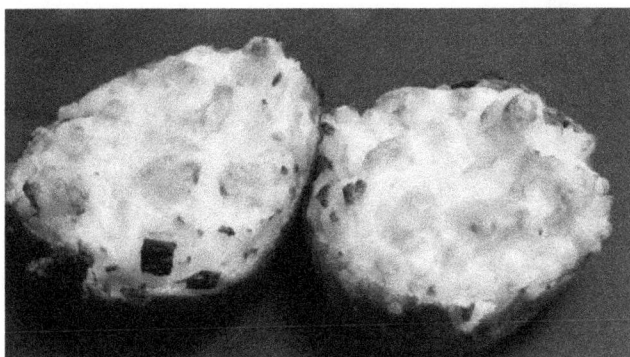

Sometimes there is nothing better than the simple things in life. A good, fiber-rich baked potato makes a delicious lunch. Follow it up with a refreshing sunshine burst of orange, dripping with vitamin C, and you are all set to enjoy an active afternoon.

Ingredients

- 1 jacket potato, no bigger than your fist
- 2 tbsp. low-fat cottage cheese
- Plus, 1 orange for afterwards

Method

1. Pre-heat the oven to 350°F. Stab the potato several times with a sharp knife, so that it cooks right through. It may take around an hour. TIP – it you are short for time, soften the potato first in a microwave by placing on high for 10 minutes.

2. When the skin of the potato is crispy and browned, then remove. Cut the potato nearly in half and top with the low-fat cottage cheese. Ready to serve this dish, which is high in fiber and high on satisfaction. Enjoy an all-natural dessert of orange segments.

Bean Crunch

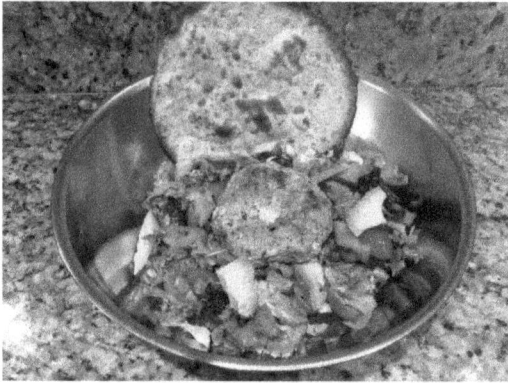

This is a tasty dish with a difference. Bean salad is delicious and filling, but high-protein pulses tend to get left off the menu far too often. This easy to prepare dish is simple and straightforward, marrying the rich textures and flavors of beans with creamy hummus and crispy, crunchy rice cakes. This recipe, once again, has two parts. If you are crazy busy, you can simply go to a deli near your office and take away 4oz of bean salad. However, you are taking a bit of a risk as it may be too heavy in terms of added olive oil, or even additives. Why not take an extra 5 minutes and play it safe by making our delicious bean salad yourself? You are guaranteed bags of low-calorie flavor and can control the levels of fat. The recipe below makes more than you will need for one meal, but it keeps for days and tastes even better after a short spell in the fridge.

Ingredients

- 4oz quick homemade bean salad
- 2 rice cakes, topped
- Low-fat hummus
- Plus 1 apple

To make the bean salad

- 1 x 14 oz. (400g) can of organic mixed beans
- 1 small onion, finely chopped
- 3 tbsp. white wine vinegar
- ½ tbsp. light olive oil
- A handful or flat-leaf parsley, finely chopped

Method

1. Drain the can of beans and pour them into a medium bowl. Add the onions to the beans and mix. In another bowl, mix the white wine vinegar and the olive oil, whipping with a fork to form a light vinaigrette emulsion. Scatter the chopped parsley over the beans and onions, then pour over the vinaigrette. Season to taste and mix well with a fork, then, if you have time, let the salad sit for at least 10 minutes to deepen the flavors.

To make the Bean Crunch

1. Lay the rice cakes on a plate and spread them thinly with low-fat hummus. Top the rice cakes with bean salad – pile

them high, it's all good! Enjoy with a large glass of water and the apple for afterwards.

Tasty Turkey Wrap

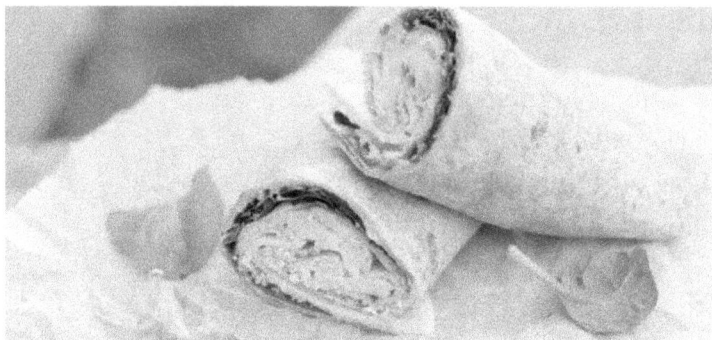

Turkey is a delicious source of lean protein that all too often gets forgotten until the holiday season. Make the most of the protein-packed goodness in this superb light lunch which brings together calcium-rich goat cheese, iron-rich spinach, plus all the protein, folate and weight-loss enhancing fiber in hummus. So many good flavors and textures, it makes for the perfect weekday lunch.

Ingredients

- 1 whole-wheat wrap
- 3 slices deli turkey
- 2 tablespoons hummus
- 1 tablespoon low-fat goat cheese
- 1 handful baby spinach

Method

1. Warm the whole-wheat wrap (optional). Spread the wrap with the hummus, lay over with turkey slices. Top with goat cheese and scatter over the baby spinach. Eat warm.

Dinner Recipes

A delicious dinner is a wonderful thing and just because you may be on a weight loss plan, there is absolutely no reason why you can't fully enjoy it! A week is not long, but far too long to eat dull, tasteless dinners. At the same time, after a busy day we do not all want to be cooking for hours, especially when we don't want to be thinking about food all the time – dinner should be simple, nutritious and enjoyable. These dinners get the balance just right.

This chapter will tell you how to prepare dinners that offer a range of different and interesting flavors. There are plenty of vegetables and some lean protein, alongside light portions of carbohydrates – all the elements of a great healthy supper. One important piece of advice should be heeded though when it comes to dinner. Do try not to eat late at night, ideally not after 7pm. After this time, the body slows down and prepares for the night sleep. When you go to sleep you meal may not be fully digested and the food sits there, plus your sluggish body take the cue to start laying down reserves of fat instead of burning of the food through exercise, for example.

Late-night eating will not help your cause, so if you tend to eat a late dinner, try bringing it forward to earlier in the evening – the habit may hopefully stick beyond 7 days. You are likely to want to try all 7 dinner recipes on offer, but do not feel tied to it – you are free to repeat your favorites during the week if you like. However, if you do enjoy all 7 dinners during the week, you will benefit from a great variety of essential nutrients. Plus remember, they are all wonderfully low in calories and fat, so tuck in without guilt and look forward to losing even more weight as you go!

Lemon Salmon

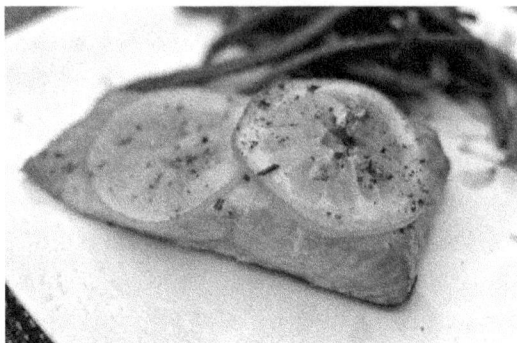

Salmon is a delicious oily fish that nutritionists love, thanks to its richness in omega-3 essential fatty acids. The delicious pink flesh is low calorie and goes beautifully with a burst of fresh, Vitamin C-packed lemon. The vegetables offer every possible combination of vitamins and minerals, depending on which you choose. Try a few of these, chopped into bite-sized pieces – broccoli, peppers, carrots, spring onions, mushrooms... or any vegetable you fancy that is not too starchy. Cook them to the degree of doneness you like, but leaving them on the crunchy side will help retain their nutrients.

Ingredients

- 1 medium salmon fillet
- Juice of 1 lemon
- 3 1/2oz mixed vegetables
- 1tsp olive oil

Method

1. Preheat the oven to 180°C. Squeeze lemon over the salmon and wrap it in foil, then bake it for about 12mins.

2. As it cooks, take a small wok or skillet and stir-fry the vegetables in the olive oil. When both the salmon and the vegetables are ready, serve and enjoy.

Tomato and Herb Chicken

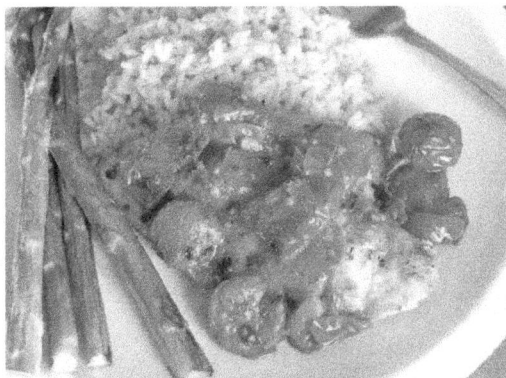

The delicious lean protein of chicken goes perfectly with the fruity goodness of tomatoes in this dish. The broccoli is ultra-low in calories, but full of fiber and nutrients. The carrots are fabulous too, sweet in taste and also full of fiber, plus carotene, which helps to ward off a wide range of diseases including heart disease. The vegetables are full of vitamins, which will support you as you lose weight and the steaming will retain more nutrients than boiling. Warming and earthy, this dish will fill you up nicely and is deceptively low in calories.

Also, don't forget you can enjoy a couple of delicious plums afterwards - they are rich in bone-healthy Vitamin K and taste great too.

Ingredients

- 1 chicken fillet
- A small tin of plum tomatoes
- 2 tsp. mixed dried herbs
- 2 ¼ oz. broccoli
- 2 ¼ oz. carrots
- Plus, 2 plums for dessert.

Method

1. Pre-heat the oven to 190°C. Place the chicken breast in an ovenproof dish. Break up the plum tomatoes a little with a fork and pour them over the chicken. Sprinkle over the dried herbs, mixing them in a little with the fork. Place the chicken and tomato dish in the oven and cook for 15-20mins.

2. When the chicken is nearly ready, cut the broccoli into florets and chop the carrot then steam over boiling water in a colander, or in a special steamer, if you have one. Ensure the chicken is cooked through with no pink and serve it in the sauce with the vegetables, when they are tender.

Sausages and Sweet Potato Mash

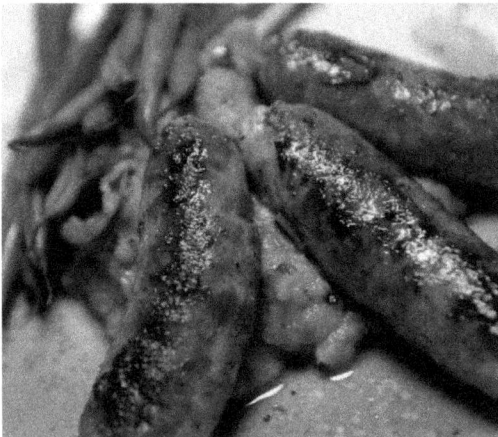

Sausages, on a diet? Yes, sure! This lovely dish combines the best type of comfort food with bags of flavor and it will all help you lose weight too – a great win-win! The sausages to use in this dish are the best quality lean beef sausages that you can find. This will keep the fat levels down to a minimum, without reducing taste.

Sweet potato is a healthier option for slimmers than normal white potato. It is higher in fiber and lower in calories and carbohydrates,

310

so it makes a great choice. Even the crème fraiche, which makes the sweet potato mash feel silky and luxurious, is another calcium-rich, low-fat version.

Ingredients

- 2 lean beef sausages
- 4oz green beans
- 1oz sweet potato
- 1tsp low-fat crème fraiche

Method

1. Preheat the grill to a medium high heat and place the sausages under it to cook, turning occasionally for 15-20 minutes. Cut the sweet potato into cubes and place in a pan of water to boil for 15 minutes or until tender.

2. When the sausages and sweet potato are nearly ready, wither place a small colander over the boiling water, place the green beans in and steam for 3 or 4 minutes, or use a steamer until they are just tender.

3. Drain the sweet potato and mash in the pan using a potato masher. Stir the teaspoon of crème fraiche into the sweet potato. Serve the sausages, with the scoop of sweet potato mash and the green beans while still hot.

Lamb Chop with Summer Veg

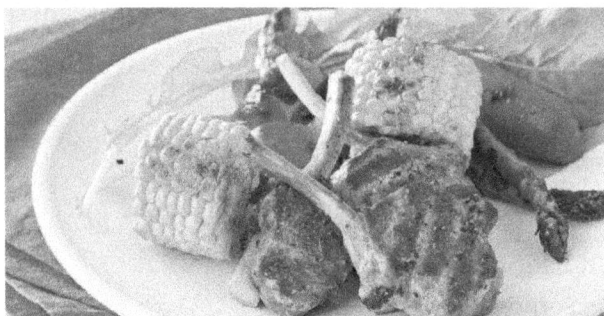

Lamb is a delicious red meat that you may have thought was "off-limits" as you drop a dress size in 7 Days. Some people find it to be fatty meat, but this depends on the way you prepare it – it certainly doesn't have to be. Happily, we know how to cook is so it remains low in fat and calories and high in protein – grilled, with as little fat as possible. Just steam some sugar snap peas, for plenty of vitamin K, A and folic acid, plus corn and serve alongside the lamb for a simple, flavorful dish.

Ingredients

- 1 small lamb chop
- 2 ¼ oz. sugar snap peas
- 2 ¼ oz. corn

Method

1. Trim the lamb of any excess fat if your butcher has not done this for you. It will still taste great and your body will thank you for it!

2. Place the chop under a medium-high grill for 10-12 minutes or until done to your liking. Steam the sugar snap peas and sweet corn by placing in a metal colander over a pan of boiling water for 3-4 minutes. Serve the hot chop and vegetables, with just a little black pepper to taste if you fancy.

Chicken Stir-Fry with Noodles

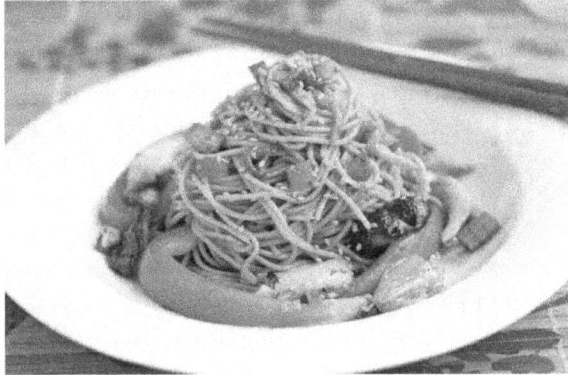

Chicken is a regular, high protein, low-fat slimmer's favorite but don't feel that you have to have it just plain grilled. This tasty stir fry packs so much color and flavor onto your plate that you'll love filling up on all these nutrients. As a tasty, filling treat, this stir-fry is served with some delicious egg noodles for that authentic oriental taste.

Ingredients

- 1 chicken breast (no skin), cut into strips
- 4 mushrooms, sliced
- 3 cherry tomatoes, sliced in two
- A handful of sugar snap peas, sliced
- A handful of baby spinach
- 2oz of egg noodles
- 1tbsp oil

Method

1. Bring a small pan of water to the boil. When boiling, drop in the egg noodles and cook for 3-5 minutes, or until just tender. Drain and set aside.

2. Heat the oil in a wok or large skillet. When the oil is really hot, add the sliced chicken to the wok. Fry for 5-7 minutes, stirring and turning with a wooden spatula.

3. When the chicken is nearly cooked (if in doubt, test with a knife to ensure no pink is showing), add the sliced vegetables but not the spinach to the wok, stirring as they cook for 2-3 minutes.

4. Before the vegetables start to go too soft – they should retain a little 'bite' - add the cooked noodles and spinach to the wok.

5. Turn down the heat and stir the ingredients around together for 1-2 minutes until the spinach has wilted and the noodles have picked up the flavors and warmed through again. Remove the stir-fry into a bowl and serve piping hot.

Mediterranean Cod with Wedges

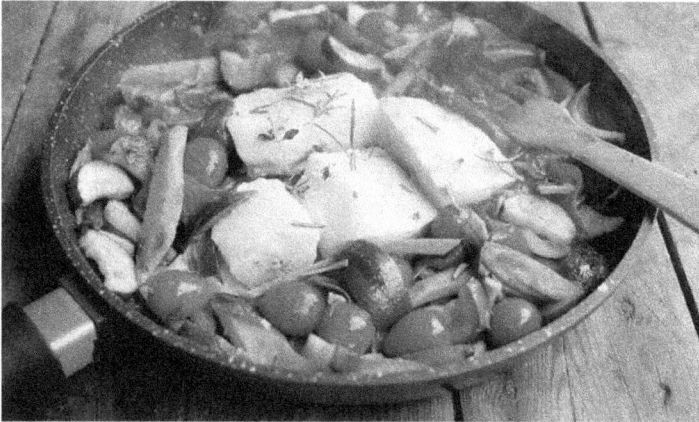

Cod is a wonderful fish. In fact, it has famously proven so popular over the years that the availability of stocks have been called into question, but happily much has been done to assure more sustainable cod is available, so buy some good quality cod to enjoy whenever you wish. It is a primary source of super-lean protein, vitamin B12, iodine and selenium plus many more nutrients. This particular dish is very tasty, thanks to the tomato-based sauce and crispy, lower-carb sweet potato wedges.

The kale is an excellent addition to your plate - full of calcium, antioxidants and super-healthy, purifying compounds, so don't miss out, it will help weight come off!

Ingredients

- 1 chunky cod fillet (or another white flaky fish, such as Pollack)
- 1 onion, chopped
- 400g can chopped tomatoes
- A few sprigs thyme, leaves stripped
- 3 oz. kale, chopped
- ½ small sweet potato
- 1 tbsp. low sodium soy sauce
- 1 tbsp. olive oil

Method

1. Preheat the oven to 180°C. Peel the sweet potato and slice into finger-sized wedges. Drizzle lightly with half the olive oil and place on a baking tray. Put into the oven for 20 minutes.

2. Meanwhile, heat the remaining olive oil in a large skillet, add the onion, and then fry for 5-8 minutes until lightly browned. Stir in the tomatoes, thyme and soy sauce, then bring it to the boil.

3. Put a pan of water on to boil, ready for the kale. Let the sauce simmer for 5 mins, then slip the cod into the skillet as well. Cover and gently cook for 8-10 mins until the cod flakes

easily. When the cod is ready, drop the kale into the boiling water and blanch it for several seconds. Drain in a colander and put on a plate.

4. Add the sweet potato wedges onto the plate with the kale, place the cod alongside and spoon over the warm tomato and onion sauce. Ready to eat and totally delectable!

Hot and Spicy Prawn Noodles

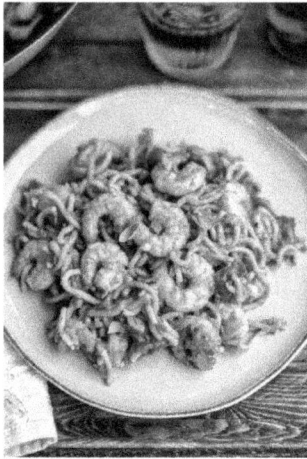

End your week (or begin it, as you prefer) with a totally flavor-packed and spicy dish. This Chinese-inspired dish brings together a whole host of great, low-calorie foods, all served up in one bowl. Prawns, which are a good source of protein and omega-3 fatty acids, lycopene-rich tomatoes, iron-rich spinach, all the vitamin C in the sweet juice and many more vitamins and nutrients besides in this low-fat dish.

Ingredients

- 2 oz. egg noodles
- 4 oz. cooked king prawns, defrosted if frozen
- ¼ large cucumber

- 2 scallions, finely sliced
- 6-8 cherry tomatoes, halved
- 1 green chili, deseeded, finely chopped
- 2 large handfuls of baby spinach leaves
- 4 tbsp. low-calorie sweet chili sauce
- 1 low sodium vegetable bouillon cube
- Zest and juice of 1 lime
- 4/5 roasted cashews, crushed

Method

1. Boil a pan of water and add the vegetable bouillon cube and stir to make stock. Add the noodles to the boiling stock for 4 mins, then drain and set aside.

2. Warm the prawns in a small skillet for a minute or two, then turn off the heat. Slice the cucumber lengthways into thick matchsticks. Add to the noodles with the scallions, tomatoes, chili and hot prawns.

3. In a small bowl, place the lime zest, juice and chili sauce and mix with a fork to make a dressing. Fold the dressing through the noodles. Put a handful of spinach onto each serving plate, top with the prawn noodles sprinkle the crushed cashews over the top.

Snack Options

So, we have run through all the great-tasting meals that you will be able to enjoy at breakfast, lunch and dinner. Now it is time to pick and choose what you fancy from the snack options available. These snacks are all healthy, low-calorie and low in fat, just like the main meal. They are wholesome and full of helpful nutrients that will encourage your body to work at its best.

Plus, by enjoying a snack twice a day, remember – you will ensure that your metabolism works at its peak function. That means burning calories even faster, so keep eating your snacks to keep losing weight!

Sounds great, right? Well, it really is that simple – just follow the plan and you will certainly lose weight. All you have to do now is pick 2 favorite snacks each day from the following 14 suggestions. Enjoy!

Cheesy Oatcakes

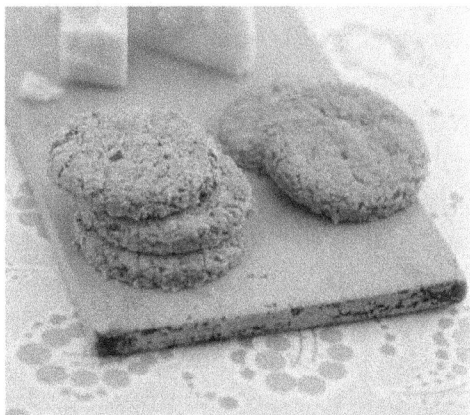

This is a quick, fun and surprisingly filling snack. Oatcakes are a fantastic form of healthy-healthy, slow-burning carbs. They contain excellent fiber and leave you feeling fuller for longer. Traditionally partnered with cheese, this low-fat cottage cheese gives you taste without the calories.

Ingredients

- 3 organic oatcakes
- 2 tbsp. reduced-fat cottage cheese
- 1 tsp. chives, finely chopped (optional)

Method

1. Take the two oatcakes and lay them on a plate. Top each oatcake with 1 tablespoon of low-fat cottage cheese. If you like, sprinkle the chopped chives over the cheese, then eat.

Crudités and Hummus

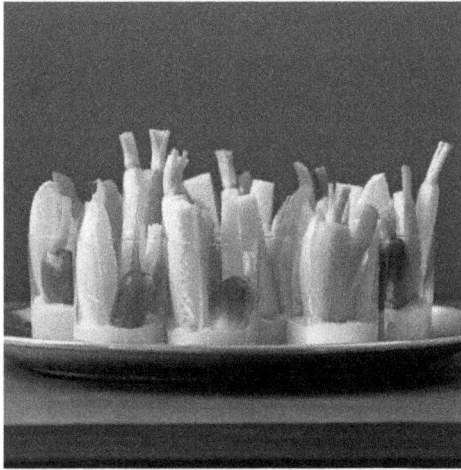

This is a great snack to tuck into when you are keen to eat something fresh-tasting and filling. Raw vegetables are simply fantastic snacks; the best nature has to offer. They offer the highest levels of nutrients, as some gets lost when you cook your veg. Add to them some creamy, chickpea-based hummus and you have a super snack that is worthy of the name.

Ingredients

- ½ cucumber
- 1 large carrot
- 2 sticks celery
- 8 radishes
- 1 tbsp. reduced-fat hummus

Method

1. Chop the cucumber across in half, so you now have two quarters, the slice the quarters lengthways, so you end up with fat matchsticks of cucumber, about the thickness of a little finger. Repeat with the carrot, chopping it into similar size matchsticks. Repeat as you chop the celery. Chop each radish in half.

2. Arrange all the vegetables on a large plate in their groups. Leave a good gap in the center. Into the gap spoon the tablespoon of reduced fat hummus. To enjoy the crudités, simply pick a piece of veg and use the hummus as a healthy dip.

Quick Veggie Broth

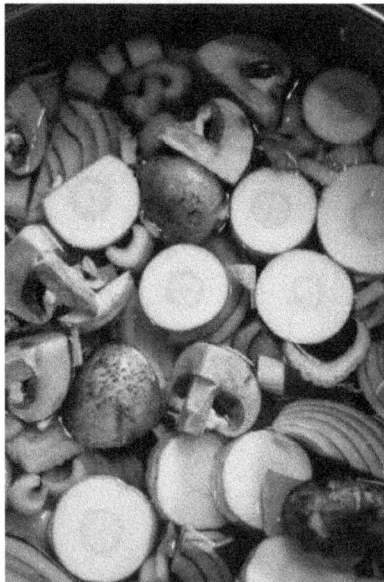

On a cold day you might want a hot snack that will warm you up without piling on the calories, especially if you have had one of the light breakfast options. Make this simple, light broth with a few vegetables. It basically just lots of fiber, water and nutrients, and it's really filling and delicious. You can make larger amounts and store some in the fridge for another snack time or to reheat at the office.

Ingredients

- 1 cup water
- 1 large carrot
- 2 celery stalks
- 4 broccoli florets, chopped into small florets
- ½ onion
- 8 mushrooms, quartered
- 1 organic chicken stock cube
- 2 sprigs of fresh parsley

Method

1. Bring the water to the boil in a pan. Toss in an organic chicken stock cube, reduce to a simmer and stir until it dissolves. Chop 1 large carrot, some broccoli florets, a few mushrooms and two celery stalks, then slice the onion into rings and add them to the stock.

2. Simmer for 5 minutes until the vegetables are tender and the stock has reduced a little, then remove to a bowl. Season with pepper, tear the parsley and scatter it over the broth then, serve.

Crackerels

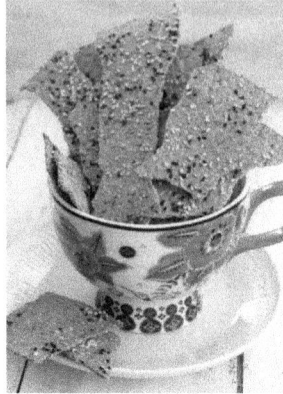

This is a fishy mid-afternoon treat, great for if you have just worked out or are planning a busy day. Mackerel is an under-used oily fish that has super levels of essential fatty acids. It goes brilliantly with cracker and here it makes the basis of a lovely fish spread, the star of a mouth-watering snack.

Ingredients

- ½ small fillet of smoked mackerel
- 2 wholegrain crackers
- 1 tbsp. fat-free plain yogurt
- 1 sprig parsley
- Freshly ground black pepper

Method

1. Remove any skin from the mackerel half-fillet and place it in bowl. Add the plain yogurt and mash it up the mackerel until it forms a coarse paste.

2. Lay the whole-grain cracker on a plate and top them with the healthy mackerel paté. Chop up the parsley leaves and sprinkle over the cracker and paté. Finish off with a grinding of black pepper and enjoy.

Fruit Portion

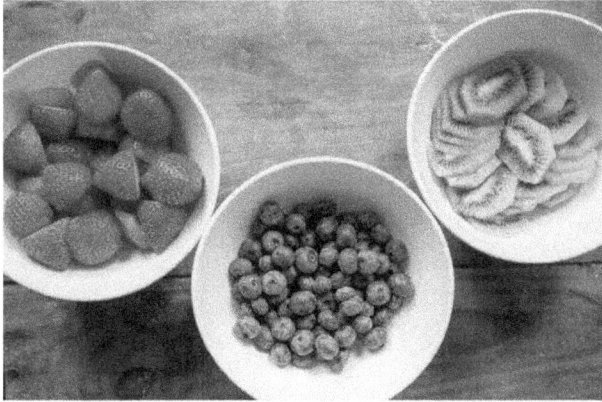

No recipe here exactly, just a hand list of good types and amounts of fruits to enjoy as a snack. This is a handy quick comparison list, since a couple of grapes will not fill you up but a whole pineapple is definitely too much! It will help you keep your calorie intake light since fruit, though delicious and healthy, does contain natural sugars, so you shouldn't fill up on it all day long and certainly not while on this plan.

Just pick a portion and enjoy it as your morning or afternoon snack:

- 1 apple
- 4 apricots
- 1 banana
- 1 cup mixed berries
- 1 cup blueberries
- 2 figs
- 1½ cups fresh fruit salad
- ½ grapefruit
- grapes
- 1 guava
- 1 kiwi fruit
- ½ mango
- 1 cup melon
- 1 orange

- 4 passion fruit
- 1 cup pawpaw
- 1 peach
- 1 pear
- 4 rings pineapple
- 2 plums
- 3 prunes
- 2 satsumas
- 1½ cup strawberries
- 1 slice watermelon

Rye Crispbread 'Pizza'

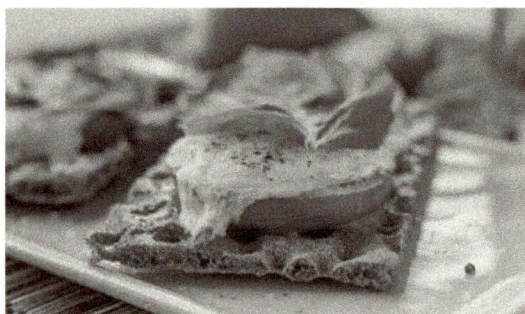

Rye crispbread are crunchy and wholesome alternatives to bread and just as versatile. They also make great snack, as is the case with this pizza-inspired low-calorie treat. Even after you have completed the plan, you might like to enjoy the occasional pair of crispbreads topped with healthy, flavorsome foods like this as a far lighter alternative to a lunchtime sandwich at your desk – they travel well.

Ingredients

- 1 rye crispbread
- 1 medium ripe tomato
- 1 tbsp. low-fat cottage cheese
- A few leaves of basil

Method

1. Lay out the rye crispbread. Top with the low-fat cottage cheese, spreading it right to the edges. Slice the tomato into medium-thick circles and place them in a layer of overlapping circles along the whole rye crispbread. Roughly tear up the basil and scatter it over your snack, then eat.

Yogurt Snack

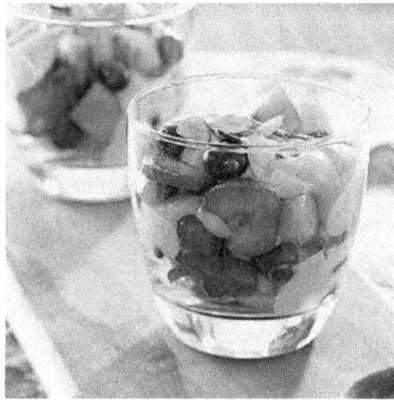

This is a fresh uncomplicated snack choice that requires no real preparation. Yogurt is a superb food for dieters. Remember the study we discussed earlier in this book, where dieters who ate some yogurt daily lost more belly fat and retained more lean muscle than those who did not eat yogurt? Great, then you will understand why this makes such a perfect snack.

Ingredients

- 150ml fat-free plain yogurt
- ½ a fruit portion from the list

Method

1. Chop your chosen fruit portion into small manageable pieces. Stir into the yogurt. Serve chilled.

Apple Chips

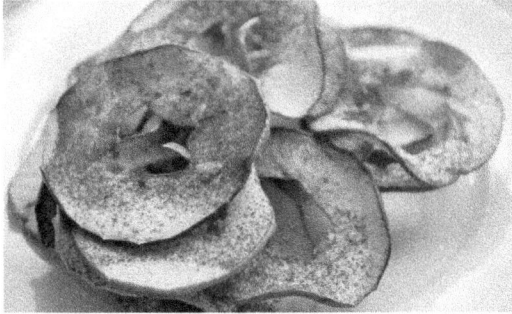

These apple chips can also be made in larger batches and stored in an airtight container for up to 3 days. They are good to take into work to enjoy when your energy levels dip during the afternoon. Don't be tempted to add any sugar to this recipe, there is enough natural fructose to give a lovely sweet and sour taste, brought out by the cinnamon. Cinnamon lowers cholesterol and reduces inflammation so do add the whole teaspoonful!

Ingredients

- 2 red apples
- 1 tsp. cinnamon

Method

1. Preheat the oven to 200 F. Thinly slice two apples crosswise about 1/8-inch (2 mm) thick with a mandolin or sharp knife.

2. Arrange apple slices in a single layer on baking sheets. Sprinkle 1 teaspoon of cinnamon evenly over apple slices. Bake for 2 hours or until apples are dry and crisp, then eat.

Kale Smoothie

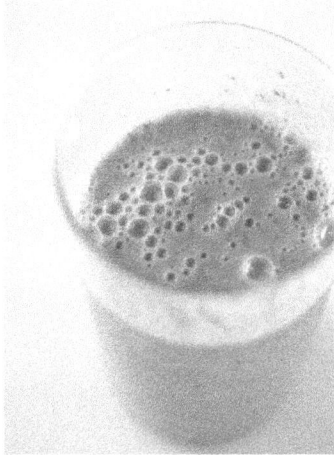

This smoothie features lots of kale, which is a dark green super-leaf. Kale is full of calcium, antioxidants and ultra-healthy, purifying compounds, which are all excellent news when you are trying to shed the toxins and the pounds. Not everyone jumps at the idea of drink a green smoothie, but the taste is softened by the apple juice and banana. Drink this when you want a shot of liquid greens – there is nothing like it for a burst of helpful nutrients.

Ingredients

- ¾ cup chopped kale, ribs and thick stems removed
- 1 stalk celery, chopped
- ½ small banana
- ½ cup unsweetened apple juice
- 1 tablespoon fresh lemon juice
- ½ cup ice

Method

1. Place the kale, celery, banana, apple juice, ice, and lemon juice in a blender. Blend until smooth and frothy then drink it nice and cold.

Popcorn Time

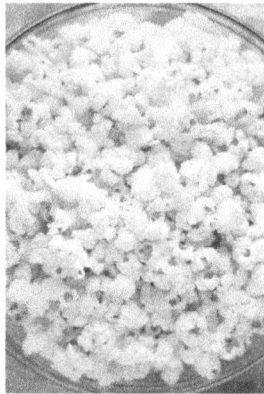

Most people are amazed when they learn how low in calories popcorn can be when it is made fresh at home. It is a very good source of fiber, so will keep you feeling full for longer, making it a top snack. Also, it's super easy to make!

Ingredients

- 20g of popping corn (just 62kcal!)
- 1 tsp. of oil

Method

1. Tip the oil into a medium-sized pan followed by the popping corn. Cover the pan with its lid – important! Heat until you hear popping, or can see the corn jumping through a glass lid.

2. Keep the heat and lid on for 1-2 minutes until the popping slows right down to the odd burst. Listening is the key – you

don't want burnt popcorn! Tip into a bowl and eat it warm.
Wonderful.

Banana Milkshake

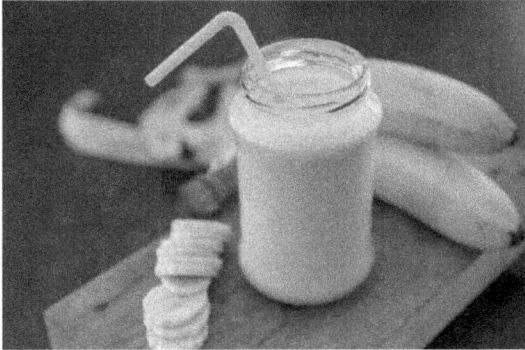

Sounds very indulgent and fattening – but of course this version
certainly isn't! Milkshakes are such a childhood treat that they can
be a hard habit to shake (excuse the pun). No need to worry though
if you use skim milk or low-fat milk. You can simply enjoy the
smooth, soothing taste as you top up your calcium levels, plus the
potassium from the banana. A snack that really hits the spot if you
have a sweet craving.

Ingredients

- 100ml low-fat milk
- 1 very ripe banana
- Ground cinnamon (optional)

Method

1. Place the banana in the blender. Top up with the milk, seal
   lid and blend fast for a few seconds until fully liquid. Pour
   the natural banana shake into a tall glass and dust the top
   with cinnamon if you like, before drinking.

Apple and Nut butter

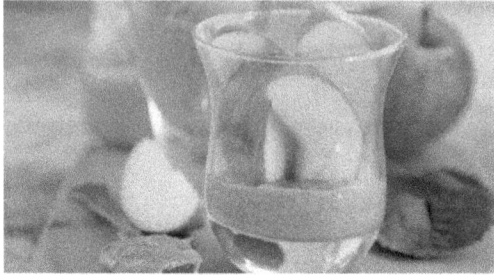

It you are after something earthy, crunchy and different from plain fruit, this combination can make a terrific treat. We know that nut butter is not low fat in large quantities, but here you are only enjoying a small amount. Why not go for walnut or almond as a healthier alternative to peanut butter – they will still give you some good, healthy omega-3 and omega-6 fatty acids. Pick a crisp, red or pink apple variety, like Pink Lady for added sweetness and crunch.

Ingredients

- 1 red apple
- 1 tsp. of nut butter

Method

1. Slice up the apple into slim wedges and enjoy a dab of nut butter with each slice – so simple, so good.

Finally... 3 Super-Fast, No-Prep Snacks

Here are a few more ideas that take no preparation whatsoever, perfect for your busiest days.

A cereal bar – A great snack for when you are always on the move. Go for a recommended brand from the health food aisle and check that it is not loaded with added sugar, glucose, corn syrup or other calorific sweeteners.

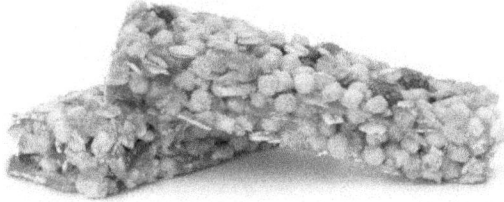

Miso soup – The packets of this savory Japanese broth are available from good health stores and supermarkets. Just empty a sachet into a mug and top up with boiling water. An incredibly low-calorie snack at around 28 calories.

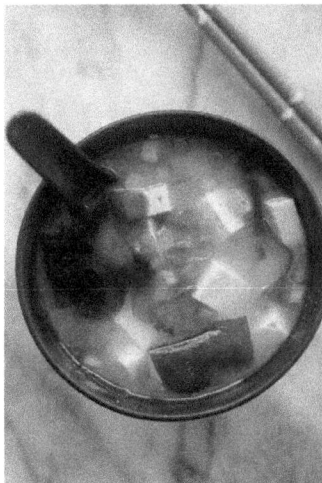

Dark chocolate – Just *three* squares of the best quality stuff you can find, don't get carried away!

Chocolate works wonders for the mood and immunity as it releases feel-good hormone serotonin into the brain and gut. Just what the doctor ordered!

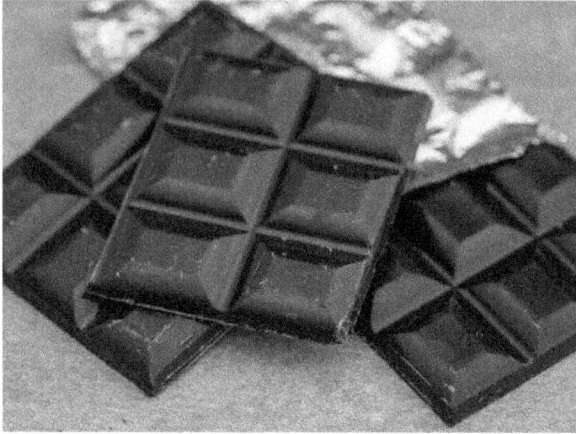

Including these quick options, that makes 14 great, very varied snacks to choose from - 2 per day for your week on the plan. Mix them up so you don't get bored of the same ones and so that you enjoy more nutrients. They are fun and good to eat – plus they WILL help you in your quest to lose weight, so enjoy.

Shopping List

Here's a shopping list with all the ingredients you need for this plan, for your convenience. The main amounts are mostly stated but not always when it comes to fruit and veg, especially as some people will want to repeat recipes and skip others. However, we recommend that you only buy the smallest amounts as it is only for 1 week.

Cereal

Box of unsweetened muesli
Cereal bars

Milk, dairy and eggs

Half a pint of semi-skimmed milk
Natural yogurt

Reduced-fat cream cheese
Reduced-fat feta
Reduced-fat mozzarella
Reduced-fat goat cheese
Low-fat yogurt
Low-fat cottage cheese
Low-fat crème fraiche
Low-fat sour cream
Free-range eggs

Fruit

Fresh raspberries
Fresh strawberries
Oranges
Plums
Apples, red
Bananas
Lemons
Limes

PLUS fruits portions of your choice

Drinks

Unsweetened orange juice

Bread Rye crispbreads

Whole-wheat bagel
Whole-meal bread, 1 loaf
Whole-grain crackers
Whole-wheat pita
Whole-meal rolls
Wholegrain tortilla

Vegetables/salad

Box of cherry tomatoes
Bag of rocket
Tomatoes
Avocado
Broccoli
Carrots
Corn
Cucumber
Gem Lettuce
Green beans
Kale
Mushrooms
Onion
Large potato for baking
Radishes
Red pepper
Scallions
Baby spinach
Sweet potatoes
Sugar snap peas
Zucchini
Oil-free salad dressing

Meat and fish

2 lean beef sausages
1 chicken breast
1 chicken fillet
1 cod fillet
Packet of lean ham
Packet of king prawns, raw
Small packet of king prawns, cooked
1 lamb chop
1 smoked mackerel fillet

1 medium salmon fillet
1 packet lean turkey breast slices

Tinned or prepared items

Small tub of low-fat hummus
Small tin of mixed beans
Small tin of plum tomatoes
Small tin of sweet corn
Small jar sun-dried tomatoes

Pasta

Egg noodles

Soups

Fresh vegetable soup (optional)
Miso soup sachet

Biscuits and snacks

Dark chocolate bar
Cashew nuts
Nut butter of choice
Oatcakes
Popping corn

Herbs, Spices and Store Cupboard Staples

Arugula
Balsamic vinegar
Basil
Chili peppers, red and green
Chives

Cinnamon
Garlic
Ginger
Ground Coriander
Hot sauce
Jar of clear honey
Low-calorie cooking spray
Olive oil (for cooking)
Mint
Mixed dried herbs
Parsley
Soy sauce, reduced sodium
Stock cubes, chicken, vegetable
Sweet chili sauce, low-calorie
Thyme
Turmeric Root
White wine vinegar
Wholegrain mustard

Discover Scientifically-Proven "Shortcuts" & "Hacks" to Lose Weight FASTER (With Very Little Effort)

For this month only, you can get Linda's best-selling & most popular book absolutely free – *Weight Loss Secrets You NEED to Know.*

Get Your FREE Copy Here:

TopFitnessAdvice.com/Bonus

Discover scientifically-proven tips to help you lose weight faster and easier than ever before. With this book, readers were able to improve their weight loss results and fitness levels. So, it's highly recommended that you get this book, especially while it's free!

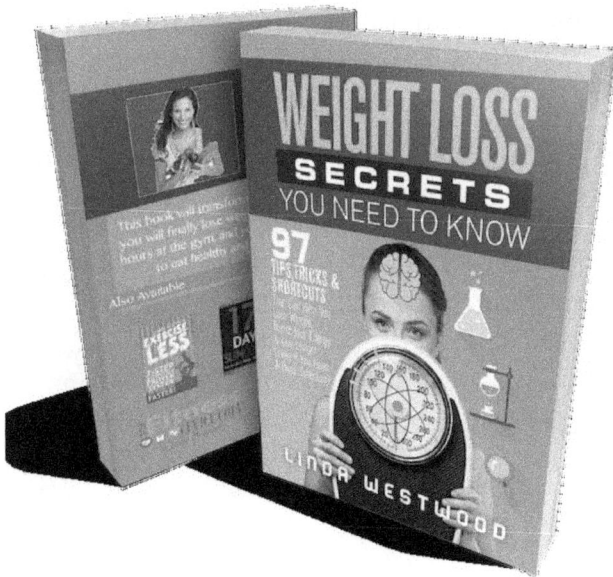

Get Your FREE Copy Here:

TopFitnessAdvice.com/Bonus

Conclusion

Very well done. Your 7 days are over and you are likely you are have undergone a radical change in eating and exercise patterns – time to enjoy the result!

This plan can do so much for your looks and health in just a week. By following the plan the majority of people will have boosted your intake of nutrients while lowering your intake of calories, leaving you better nourished than you may have been in a while… but at the same time, much lighter!

Take a look in the mirror now. Chances are you are looking slimmer, with brighter eyes and more glowing skin, especially is you stuck to drinking lots of water throughout the week as advised.

You should congratulate yourself on having achieved considerable internal benefits too – better digestion, fewer toxins in your system, less strain on your joints, heart and organs and a reduced risk of diseases, all of which come with losing weight the healthy way, with exercises included.

You will have speeded up your metabolism, gained in strength and flexibility, and increased tone in your muscles all over, including in the leg, butt and abdomen area…

But most obviously of all, for all of these reasons you will be **looking and feeling great!** In just 7 days you have effected a transformation inside and out and that is worth celebrating.

Remember:

You stuck to a healthy diet plan and did not starve yourself, eating every 3-4 hours and enjoying snacks.

You carried out a tailor-made exercise plan, without all the usual reps, for toning and smoothing muscles plus burning calories

You have done all you can to accelerate the weight loss process, from drinking water and staying off the alcohol, to sleeping properly and trying detoxifying treats like saunas.

Of course, you know exactly how you need to celebrate it...

Why not go to the wardrobe now and try on that size smaller dress?

You deserve to feel the benefits of your change and it will remind you of how far you have come in a relatively short time.

As dresses may not be as precise every time, you should also measure your inches too and write them down in the dedicated spaces in Chapter 2, just so you can compare them with your 'Before' stats - an exciting moment!

But back to that special dress, if you have one.

If you were always planning to wear it to a party or wedding, or on holiday, we hope you are delighted with the fact that you will look better than ever for the big occasion.

Wear it with pride as you continue to benefit from the low-fat, low-calorie diet and added exercise lifestyle improvements you have made in the past 7 days.

The new habits that you adopted in this plan are changes that, if continued, will ensure your fitness, happiness and health for long into the future.

Enjoying this book?

Check out my other best sellers!

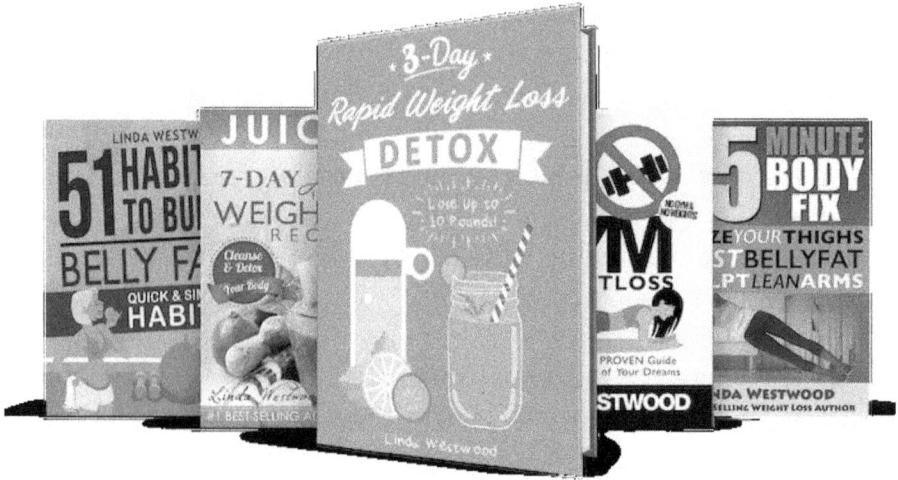

Final Words

I would like to thank you for purchasing my book and I hope I have been able to help you and educate you on something new.

If you have enjoyed this book and would like to share your positive thoughts, could you please take 30 seconds of your time to go back and give me a review on my Amazon book page.

I greatly appreciate seeing these reviews because it helps me share my hard work.

You can leave me a review on Amazon.com.

Again, thank you and I wish you all the best!

www.ingramcontent.com/pod-product-compliance
Lightning Source LLC
Chambersburg PA
CBHW031139020426
42333CB00013B/446